assessment and
investigative Techniques

D1423677

Commissioning Editor: Robert Edwards

For Elsevier Butterworth-Heinemann:

Publishing Director: Caroline Makepeace
Development Editor: Kim Benson
Project Manager: Anne Dickie
Design Direction: George Ajayi

eye essentials

assessment and investigative techniques

Sandip Doshi PhD, MCOptom
Optometrist in private practice, Hove, East Sussex, UK
Examiner, College of Optometrists, London, UK
Formerly Clinical Editor, Optician Journal

William Harvey MCOptom
*Visiting Clinician and Director of Visual Impairment Clinic, City University,
London, UK*
Professional Programme Tutor for Boots Opticians Ltd
Clinical Editor, Optician Journal, Reed Business Information, Sutton, UK

SERIES EDITORS
Sandip Doshi PhD, MCOptom
Optometrist in private practice, Hove, East Sussex, UK
Examiner, College of Optometrists, London, UK
Formerly Clinical Editor, Optician Journal

William Harvey MCOptom
Visiting Clinician and Director of Visual Impairment Clinic, City University, London, UK
Professional Programme Tutor for Boots Opticians Ltd
Clinical Editor, Optician Journal, Reed Business Information, Sutton, UK

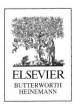

ELSEVIER
BUTTERWORTH
HEINEMANN

EDINBURGH LONDON NEW YORK OXFORD
PHILADELPHIA ST LOUIS SYDNEY TORONTO 2005

ELSEVIER
BUTTERWORTH
HEINEMANN

© 2005, Elsevier Limited. All rights reserved.
First published 2005

No part of this publication may be reproduced, stored in a retrieval system, or transmitted in any form or by any means, electronic, mechanical, photocopying, recording or otherwise, without either the prior permission of the publishers or a licence permitting restricted copying in the United Kingdom issued by the Copyright Licensing Agency, 90 Tottenham Court Road, London W1T 4LP. Permissions may be sought directly from Elsevier's Health Sciences Rights Department in Philadelphia, USA: (+1) 215 238 7869, fax: (+1) 215 238 2239, e-mail: healthpermissions@elsevier.com. You may also complete your request on-line via the Elsevier homepage (http://www.elsevier.com), by selecting 'Customer Support' and then 'Obtaining Permissions'.

ISBN 0 7506 8853 X

British Library Cataloguing in Publication Data
A catalogue record for this book is available from the British Library.

Library of Congress Cataloging in Publication Data
A catalog record for this book is available from the Library of Congress.

Note
Knowledge and best practice in this field are constantly changing. As new research and experience broaden our knowledge, changes in practice, treatment and drug therapy may become necessary or appropriate. Readers are advised to check the most current information provided (i) on procedures featured or (ii) by the manufacturer of each product to be administered, to verify the recommended dose or formula, the method and duration of administration, and contraindications. It is the responsibility of the practitioner, relying on their own experience and knowledge of the patient, to make diagnoses, to determine dosages and the best treatment for each individual patient, and to take all appropriate safety precautions. To the fullest extent of the law, neither the publisher nor the editors assumes any liability for any injury and/or damage to persons or property arising from this publication.

Working together to grow
libraries in developing countries

www.elsevier.com | www.bookaid.org | www.sabre.org

ELSEVIER   BOOK AID
            International   Sabre Foundation

ELSEVIER   your source for books,
            journals and multimedia
            in the health sciences

www.elsevierhealth.com

The
publisher's
policy is to use
**paper manufactured
from sustainable forests**

Printed in China

Contents

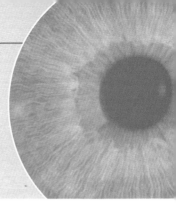

Acknowledgments

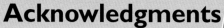

Thanks to Heidi, Tallulah, Kitty, Spike and Van der Graaf Generator

Bill Harvey

To my family, Bhauna, Jai and Kiran for their love and support, and to Snoop Dogg for all his inspiration

Sandip Doshi

Foreword

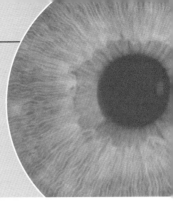

Eye Essentials is a series of books intended to cover the core skills required by the eye care practitioner in general and/or specialized practice. It consists of books covering a wide range of topics, ranging from: routine eye examination to assessment and management of low vision; assessment and investigative techniques to digital imaging; case reports and law to contact lenses.

Authors known for their interest and expertise in their particular subject have contributed books to this series. The reader will know many of them, as they have published widely within their respective fields. Each author has addressed key topics in their subject in a practical rather than theoretical approach, hence each book has a particular relevance to everyday practice.

Each book in the series follows a similar format and has been designed to enable the reader to ascertain information easily and quickly. Each chapter has been produced in a user-friendly format, thus providing the reader with a rapid-reference book that is easy to use in the consulting room or in the practitioner's free time.

Optometry and dispensing optics are continually developing professions, with the emphasis in each being redefined as we learn more from research and as technology stamps its mark. The *Eye Essentials* series is particularly relevant to the practitioner's requirements and as such will appeal to students, graduates sitting professional examinations and qualified practitioners alike. We hope you enjoy reading these books as much as we have enjoyed producing them.

Sandip Doshi
Bill Harvey

1
Vision, acuity and contrast sensitivity

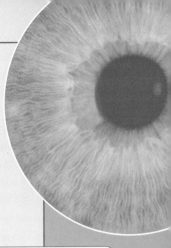

Introduction

It is both clinically and legally important to be able to record how well a patient can see. If any ocular assessment or investigation is to be undertaken, a baseline measurement of visual capability is evidence that the procedure has not caused a reduction in vision, or at least one that had not been predicted. Knowledge of the level of vision of a patient may also dictate what assessment is to be undertaken (for example in refraction, the size of dioptric steps to be presented to the patient, or the area of fundus to be examined). Over a sequence of assessments, the level of vision is a useful indication of any progression of disease or age-related change. So for any consultation, an optometrist should record at the outset, often throughout, and then at the conclusion, a record of the level of vision in each eye of the patient.

Visual acuity and vision

Visual acuity is a measurement of a patient's ability to resolve detail and usually involves directing a patient to identify targets at a set distance which are of ever-decreasing size and typically of high-contrast until they can no longer be identified. The recognition of high-contrast targets at the highest spatial frequency as described is useful for standardized assessment but is not representative of the visual environment within which the patient lives and hence will not truly represent the patient's visual ability. The unaided visual acuity (usually called the vision) is useful in estimating refractive error before assessment and represents important baseline data where a patient does not use, or perhaps does not need to use, their correction all the time. The acuity with their current correction is known as the habitual visual acuity and the resultant visual acuity after refraction and full correction of the current refractive error is known as the optimal visual acuity. It is essential for an optometrist to note either the vision or habitual visual acuity prior to any clinical assessment in case of any legal action taken as a result of the examination. Both monocular and binocular acuity should be noted as there may be a discrepancy, such as when a nystagmus patient shows significant acuity improvement when in the binocular state.

Although there are several ways to specify target size on test charts, the most widely used system was introduced by Snellen in 1862. He assumed that the 'average' eye could just read a letter if the thickness of the limbs and the spaces between them subtended one minute of arc at the eye. Thus the letter E would subtend five minutes of arc vertically. Snellen notation requires the acuity allowing the eye to resolve such a letter to be noted down as a fraction with the viewing distance (usually in meters and commonly 6 m) over the distance at which such a target would subtend 5 minutes of arc vertically. Thus at 6 m a 6/6 letter subtends five minutes of arc vertically, a 6/12 letter 10 minutes and a 6/60 letter 50 minutes. The Snellen fraction may also be written as a decimal, for example 6/6 = 1, 6/12 = 0.5 and 6/60 = 0.1.

An alternative is to record the minimum angle of resolution (MAR). The MAR relates to the resolution required to resolve the elements of a letter. Thus 6/6 equates to a MAR of 1 minute of arc, 6/12 to an MAR of 2 and 6/60 to 10. The logMAR score is the $\log_{10}$ of the MAR and so is 0 for 6/6 and 1 for 6/60. This means that targets smaller than the 6/6 letters, which would be expected to be resolved by a young healthy adult, would carry a negative score value. Some acuity values are shown in different notation in Table 1.1.

Table 1.1 **The relationship between different acuity scales**

Snellen	Decimal	MAR	LogMAR
6/60	0.10	10	1.000
6/24	0.25	4	0.602
6/12	0.50	2	0.301
6/6	1.00	1	0.000
6/4	1.50	0.667	−0.176

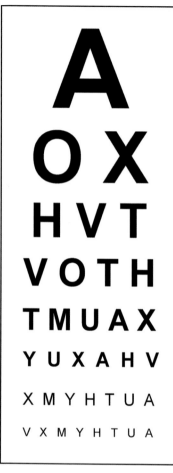

Figure 1.1 The standard Snellen chart (reproduced with permission from Doshi & Harvey *Investigative Techniques and Ocular Examination,* Butterworth-Heinemann 2003)

LogMAR notation

Though Snellen notation is still in widespread use, there are criticisms of the standard Snellen chart as shown in Figure 1.1.

There are fewer large letters so providing an unequal challenge to those with reduced vision, the letter spacing reduces leading to crowding on lower lines, the line separation is not regular so the challenge changes on reading down the chart which means that moving charts to different working distances alters the demand on acuity. LogMAR charts, such as the Bailey–Lovie chart shown in Figure 1.2, address some of these shortcomings by having spacing between letters on each line related to the width of the letters and between rows relating to the height of the letters, and an equal number of letters on each line. This provides a constant task as the patient reads down the chart allowing it to be viewed at different working distances and the acuity to be more easily correlated. Such charts have been found to give greater repeatability of measurement, when compared with standard Snellen charts, and to be more sensitive to detect interocular acuity differences.

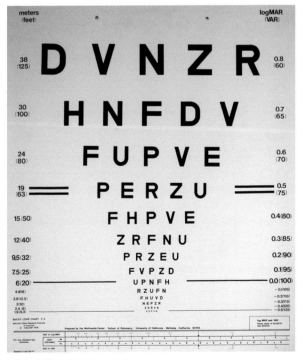

Figure 1.2 The Bailey–Lovie chart

LogMAR scores may be noted on record cards either relating to the smallest target line size seen or using the Visual Acuity Rating where 0.02 is added for every letter missed on the line. So where a patient just manages the 6/6 line and no more they are scored as 0. If they miss two letters on this line they are scored as 0.04. Until this notation becomes universally accepted, Snellen notation is still appropriate for referrals and interprofessional communication. Most logMAR charts in use are calibrated for a working distance of 4 meters.

When one has to reduce the distance, for example for a low-vision patient, it is useful to remember to add 0.3 to the score for every time the distance is halved. For example the ability to read the top line at 4 meters would be scored as acuity of 1.0. At 2 m, this would be scored as 1.3.

So if a patient with visual impairment only manages two letters of the 0.9 line on a 4-meter logMAR chart held at 2 meters, this would be noted as (0.94 + 0.3) or 1.24.

Other vision charts

Where letter recognition is not possible, for example with small children or patients of different literacy, a whole range of picture and line targets are available. Some require identification, others matching of targets with a separate key card. For the very young, the use of gratings of different spatial frequency next to blank targets may be presented to see if the infant's attention is directed to the grating. Such preferential-looking tests have been found to show good repeatability in pediatric assessment.

Near vision assessment

The Faculty of Ophthalmologists Times New Roman near chart

The Faculty of Ophthalmologists Times New Roman chart for near vision is still the most widely used in optometric practice. It offers high contrast blocks of text ranging from N48 to N5 or in some cases N4.5. The relationship of print size is easily understood. N5 is half the size of N10; N18 is three times larger than N6, etc. Whilst an accurate measurement of near acuity is arguably required for comparisons between successive visits, many patients comment that the high contrast of the print (≥90%) test card bears less resemblance to the ability to read at home. Most newsprint and paperback novels are printed in lower contrast (~75%), which is further reduced with age and use. There is also the risk of glare when the card is laminated.

Near logMAR chart

The near logMAR chart (Figure 1.3) has all the advantages of a logarithmic scale. It may test from N80 to N2 with a random selection of words, allowing improved testing of threshold near acuity. However at the larger sizes there are a limited number of words available and therefore it is unfeasible to assess the quality of a patient's reading performance with this chart.

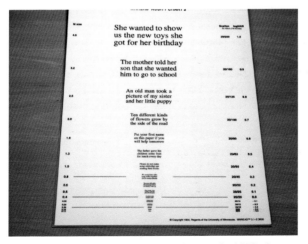

Figure 1.3   The MNRead is an example of a near logMAR chart

The Keeler A series chart

The Keeler A series chart has a logarithmic progression. In the Keeler A system the letter size labeled as A1 has lower case letters whose overall angular subtense at the test's designated standard distance of 25 cm is 5′ arc. It is used primarily in low-vision assessment (see *Low Vision Assessment* by Jane MacNaughton in this series).

MNREAD acuity charts

The Minnesota Low-Vision Reading Test is a computer-based system for measuring reading speed. This test has more recently been created as a printed card version (Figure 1.4) for use within clinical practice. The cards are printed in high contrast, including reverse contrast and print size varies from logMAR 1.3 to –0.5 (N64 to N1). The practitioner records the time taken for the patient to read a sentence of unrelated words, each of same length (60 characters, 10 standard length words) and reads down the charts until mistakes are made. The cards have been demonstrated to have significant value on the evaluation of reading performance and are becoming more widely used in low-vision clinics.

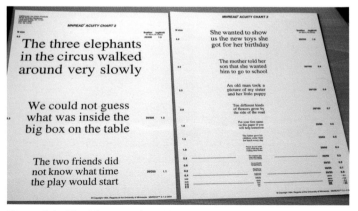

Figure 1.4 The Minnesota Low-Vision Reading Test

The McClure Reading Test

The McClure Reading Test (Figure 1.5) has been designed specifically for use with children. It contains reading material of varying difficulty or standards, appropriate for different age groups. It is important to be able to assess the child's ability to see to read rather than their ability to read, especially for those children who have difficulty reading aloud. However, one disadvantage is that the child's age group appears at the top of the printed text, and this can be off-putting for those children who are sensitive to their reading capabilities. (For a full description of targets useful for visually impaired children, see Harper R (2004) *Low Vision Assessment and Management* in Harvey & Gilmartin, *Paediatric Optometry*, Butterworth-Heinemann).

CHILDRENS READING TYPE.

age group 4-5 years

N5

N6

N8
here is a toy
the boy plays with the toy
the toy is on the red rug
the cat likes the rug
the cat plays with the boy on the rug
the boy likes to play with the cat

N10
here is a tree
the tree is wet
the ball is in the tree
I like the girl
the girl runs to the tree for the ball
the ball is big and wet

N12
here is a cat
the cat has a toy
the boy plays with the cat
the cat likes the toy
the girl and the boy play with the cat
the dog can run with the boy

N14
here is a dog
the dog can run
the girl likes the dog
the girl has fun
the dog can run for the ball
the girl and the dog have fun

age group 5-6 years

N5

N6

N8
Here is a boy and here is a big dog.
They have fun with the ball.
The ball is in the water and the
dog jumps into the water.
The dog can get the ball from the water,
but the boy can not get the fish.

N10
Here is a pig and here is a tree.
I can see the pig and the big tree.
I like to play with a ball and have fun.
Here is some water by the tree.
The pig can go to the water.
He can see a big fish in the water.

N12
Here is a girl and here is a shop.
It is a sweet shop and a toy shop.
The girl likes the toys in the shop.
She can have fun with the toys.
The girl can go to the shop to get some dolls.
She can get big toys in the shop.

N14
Here is a man and here is a cat.
The cat has fun with a toy.
They are on the red rug.
The cat can sit with the man.
We like to see the cat have fun.
The man has to go home to see the cat.

Figure 1.5   Samples from the McClure Reading Test showing print for different age groups (reproduced with permission from Harvey & Gilmartin *Paediatric Optometry*, Butterworth-Heinemann, 2004)

Relating distance to near measurements

As these measurements generally rely upon recognition of a target just large enough to be resolved, it should be possible to predict from the distance acuity exactly what the near acuity might be. A letter just seen at 6 meters should subtend the same angle at the retina as a smaller letter seen at 25 cm. This is often not the case, though in the healthy eye the prediction is rarely far wrong. However, certain disease will tend to have greater impact upon the ability to resolve targets at different distances. Posterior subcapsular cataract, for example, will tend to cause greater blur when viewing near targets. Macular degeneration results in a central scotoma which has a greater impact upon the near field of view. Nystagmus may be dampened on convergence resulting in a significantly improved acuity for near targets than for distant ones.

The scoring of a 25 cm logMAR reading chart should correlate with the distance one. So the ability to resolve the 0.6 line at 4 m should also allow the 0.6 line to be read on the 25 cm near chart, assuming that the patient is corrected for the near target.

For Snellen notation, a 'rule-of-thumb' is often adopted which aims to predict the size of N number target which will just fit into the imagined lines drawn from the top and bottom of the letter just seen at 6 meters. The N value is seen to be around one third the value of the denominator of the distance acuity. For example, distance acuity of 6/24 should correlate roughly with N8 at 25 cm, 6/18 with N6 and 3/60 (or 6/120) with N40. This prediction of the expected near visual capability is particularly useful in judging a patient's response to a near correction, especially if it entails a working distance which may initially present a challenge to the patient.

Contrast sensitivity testing

The ability to resolve targets varies significantly with the contrast of the target. The visual world a patient inhabits is one of varying target size and contrast and, furthermore, diseases affecting vision may affect the ability to resolve these targets in a selective manner. Therefore, the use of high-contrast targets for acuity testing has been criticized as unrepresentative of the visual world and less than sensitive at reflecting visual reduction due to disease. If a patient is shown a sine-wave grating of a constant spatial frequency, as shown in Figure 1.6, their ability to resolve the grating reduces as the contrast is reduced until a point is reached when it can no longer be resolved. This point, the contrast threshold (the reciprocal of which is called the contrast sensitivity), is different for different spatial frequencies and the plot of the threshold values against spatial frequency is described as the contrast sensitivity function (CSF) as shown in Figure 1.7.

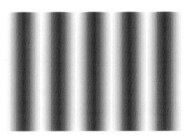

Figure 1.6 A sine-wave grating (reproduced with permission from Doshi & Harvey *Investigative Techniques and Ocular Examination*, Butterworth-Heinemann 2003)

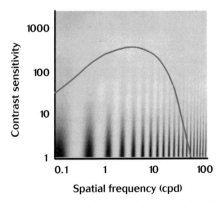

Spatial frequency (cpd)

Figure 1.7 Contrast sensitivity function (reproduced with permission from Doshi & Harvey *Investigative Techniques and Ocular Examination*, Butterworth-Heinemann 2003)

Snellen acuity relates to the resolution of a high-contrast target of maximum spatial frequency and is therefore represented as the cut-off point on the horizontal axis (as represented by the arrow in Figure 1.7) on this curve. This is sensitive to conditions affecting mainly high spatial frequencies, such as refractive error, but less sensitive if lower spatial frequencies are affected, as with cataract, corneal disturbance or contact lens wear.

Increasingly clinicians are using targets of different contrast to assess the influence upon acuity. LogMAR charts are available in different contrasts so assessing the patient's ability to resolve increasing spatial frequencies at a given contrast value. Computerized acuity charts, such as the City2000 shown in Figure 1.8, allow any contrast value to be preset.

Other charts, such as the Pelli–Robson (Figure 1.9), use a constant letter size (approximating to one cycle per degree if viewed at 1 m) and gradually reducing contrast as the chart is read by the patient. In theory, varying the working distance would allow the whole contrast sensitivity function to be assessed with

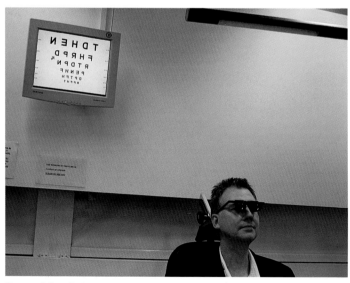

Figure 1.8 Computerized acuity chart

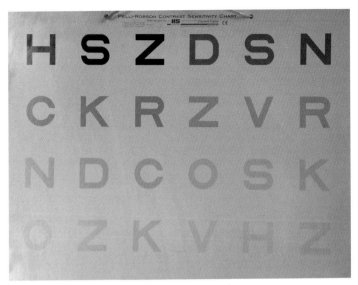

Figure 1.9 Pelli–Robson contrast sensitivity chart

a Pelli–Robson chart, but in practice this is rarely needed as high- and low-contrast acuity scores combined with contrast sensitivity at 1 m with a Pelli–Robson is usually sufficient to suggest any visual compromise.

Other contrast charts available for clinical practice include the Vistech. This is a poster with five rows of circles upon which is printed a grating. Each row represents a constant spatial frequency but, as the patient looks along the row from left to right, the contrast of the grating decreases until it is no longer possible to state in which direction the grating is orientated (to the left or to the right, for example). This way, a score representing the limit of contrast resolution for each predefined spatial frequency may be noted and plotted as a CSF curve. The test is limited, however, by the necessarily limited number of targets viewed.

Less commonly seen now are the Arden gratings. These are a sequence of cards upon which a grating of a constant spatial frequency is printed but which decreases in contrast until no longer discernible. The card is slowly moved out from a masking card (minimum contrast first) until the patient states they can first see the grating pattern revealed. This is done for each card representing a different spatial frequency and so a score may be attributed to the overall sensitivity to contrast at each.

Method of acuity testing

The following list represents some important points to bear in mind when recording acuity during an eye examination.

- Binocular followed by monocular acuity is useful. The binocular acuity is occasionally different to the monocular (for example much better in many nystagmus patients). Also this order allows an assessment of acuity prior to the breakdown of a less-stable binocular state once an occluder is introduced.
- The acuity with current spectacles is useful as it represents the patient's actual experience. It is important therefore to simulate as closely as possible the typical viewing conditions for the patient (usually with the room lights on).
- If one eye is known to have poorer vision, this should be assessed first to minimize any learning of targets.
- An occluder should be used and checked for correct placement. Use of hands should be avoided as often the patient may see through a gap between fingers not apparent to anyone else.
- Any indication of the quality of the acuity should be noted together with the notation for the minimum target size seen (for example 'blurred 6/12-1, or 6/48 viewed eccentrically).
- For distance acuity, note should be made of the correction being worn and its condition.
- For near acuity, a target distance relating to the patient's everyday experience (computer or reading distance) should be adopted. For near vision, the distance at which the best vision is achieved gives some clues about the uncorrected refractive error and this should be noted.
- When uncorrected vision is poor, it is better to attempt some sort of quantification rather than rely upon imprecise

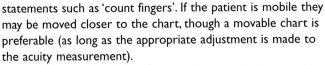
statements such as 'count fingers'. If the patient is mobile they may be moved closer to the chart, though a movable chart is preferable (as long as the appropriate adjustment is made to the acuity measurement).

- If a patient is to be referred, a note of the acuity is essential, even in the case of an emergency referral such as of a retinal detachment.

Finally, almost all of the preceding methods of assessing acuity and vision have some subjective element in that they rely upon the patient reporting what they can make out of a target. For this reason, it is often very useful to also make a note of the quality of the image a patient has. If they can just about see a letter, or if the middle of a row of letters may only be seen by looking at the end of the row, then a note of this may be useful when later giving advice to the patient on their level of vision.

2
Investigation of color vision

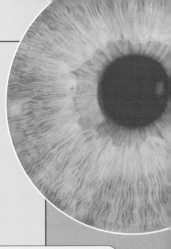

Introduction

Assessment of color vision is an integral part of any eye examination. Congenital color defects have a high prevalence, particularly among males, and have an impact upon visual interpretation and career demands. Furthermore, color deficiency may be acquired as a result of disease or drug and toxin effects and screening for such is an important part of ocular health assessment.

Inheritance, prevalence and molecular genetics of inherited deficiency

Types of inherited color vision deficiencies

Color deficiency is caused by inherited photopigment abnormalities and as such there are three different types in man. These vary in severity within each subgroup. Some colors that look markedly different to people with normal color vision appear to be the same to color-deficient patients and consequently may be confused. Relative color lightness and contrast are also changed as a result of an alteration in the relative luminous efficiency of the eye. Colors are confused when there are no perceived lightness differences.

Normal trichromatic color vision in man is derived from the three types of cone photopigment. These have a maximum sensitivity around 420, 530 and 560 nm. Three color-matching variables are needed to match all the spectral hues. The terms used to describe different types of color deficiency are based on the number of photopigments present and hence the number of color-matching variables needed. The majority of color-deficient patients have three photopigments, but the spectral sensitivity of one photopigment is abnormal. In fewer people one, two or all of the photopigments may be lacking or abnormal (Table 2.1).

Monochromats may be described as typical or atypical. In the former, also referred to as rod-monochromats, there are no

Table 2.1 Classification of inherited color vision deficiencies

Number of cone photopigments	Type	Denomination	Hue-discrimination ability
None	Monochromat	Typical (rod) monochromat	None
One	Monochromat	Atypical, 'incomplete' monochromat	Limited discrimination in mesopic conditions
Two	Dichromat	Protanope Deutranope Tritanope	Severely impaired
Three	Anomalous trichromat	Protanomalous Deutranomalous Tritanomalous	Slight to severe impairment

functioning cones. Consequently, acuity is poor, typically around 6/60–6/36. These patients are photophobic and have nystagmus. The lack of cones results in no cone-mediated responses, however, in rare cases, cone photopigments are present but the lack of color vision results from an abnormality in the visual pathway. Atypical 'incomplete' monochromats have the photopigment sensitive to short wavelengths only. Some color discrimination is possible in mesopic conditions, when both rods and cones are functioning. Visual acuity is reduced, but not as much as in typical form, tending to range between 6/24–6/9. Photophobia and nystagmus are only present in those with acuity less than 6/18.

The term protan, deutan and tritan are derived from the Greek words meaning first, second and third. These are terms used to describe color deficiency that involves a particular type of photopigment. Each term includes dichromatism and anomalous trichromatism. Both protans and deutans make similar color confusions in the red–yellow–green part of the spectrum. These colors are used in pseudoisochromatic screening to

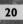

identify both types of red–green color deficiency. Achromatic or 'neutral' colors, which are confused with gray, are different in protans and deutans and these colors are used in pseudoisochromatic designs to distinguish or classify, protan and deutan color deficiency. Dichromats confuse bright, fully saturated colors while anomalous trichromats confuse pale, less-saturated colors (see Table 2.2).

Table 2.2 **Colors confused by protan, deutan and tritan color deficiency**

| | Type of color deficiency | | |
Color confusion	Protan	Deutan	Tritan
Red/orange/yellow/green	*	*	
Brown/green	*	*	
Green/white threshold saturation discrimination	*	*	
Red/white threshold saturation discrimination	*	*	
Blue–green/gray/red–purple	*		
Green/gray/blue–purple		*	
Red/black	*		
Green/black		*	
Violet/yellow–green			*
Red/red–purple			*
Dark blue/black			*
Yellow/white			*

Prevalence of inherited color vision deficiency

Population studies show the prevalence of red–green color deficiency to be around 8% in men and 0.4% in women. There is therefore an X-chromosome relationship to color deficiency.

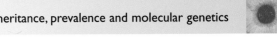
A large study carried out in 1975 confirmed that deutranomalous trichromatism was the most common type of color deficiency (see Table 2.3).

Table 2.3 **Approximate prevalence of red–green color deficiency**

Type of color deficiency	Prevalence in men (%)	Prevalence in women (%)
Protanopia	1	0.01
Protanomalous trichromatism	1	0.03
Deutranopia	1	0.01
Deutranomalous trichromatism	5	0.35
Total prevalence	8	0.40

Prevalence of color vision deficiency is not thought to vary with ethnicity, geographic latitude or cultural development. The prevalence of genetic disorders is always different in populations that are isolated geographically or by religious practice because the gene pool is restricted. Geographic isolation and intermarriage between people who share a common ancestor is responsible for the high prevalence of typical rod-monochromatism.

Congenital tritan defects are inherited as autosomal dominant trait and there is an equal prevalence between men and women. The frequency of congenital tritanopia is very low, typically in the order of 1 in 10 000; however, the prevalence of tritanomalous trichromatism may be as high as 1 in 500.

Inheritance and genetics

In each generation there are four possible combinations of X and Y chromosomes that children inherit from their parents (see Figure 2.1). All daughters from a color-deficient father inherit his X chromosome with the gene anomaly and are carriers of the color deficiency. They transmit the same abnormal chromosome to 50% of their sons, who are color deficient, and 50% to their

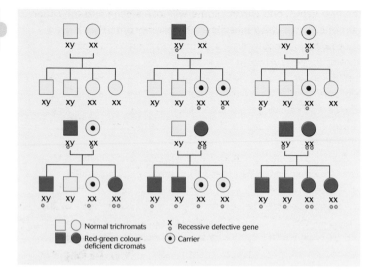

Figure 2.1 Examples of X-linked inheritance (reproduced with permission from Doshi & Harvey *Investigative Techniques and Ocular Examination*, Butterworth-Heinemann 2003)

daughters, who are carriers. Brothers of a color-deficient man have a 50% risk of being similarly affected. Women are only color deficient if they inherit abnormal X chromosome genes for the same photopigment from both parents. Women who are mixed-compound heterozygotes (carriers), with an abnormal gene coding for a protan defect on one X chromosome and for a deutan defect on the other have normal color vision.

Long- and medium-wavelength photopigment genes are positioned in a tandem 'head-to-tail' array near the end of the long (q) arm of the X chromosome (Xq28) and have almost identical amino-acid sequences. Both genes consist of 264 amino acids and differ at only 15 sites. This suggests that the two genes evolved from a single gene sensitive to middle waves fairly recently in the evolutionary timescale. The close proximity and similarity of the photopigment genes means that crossover of genetic material can occur during meiosis. If the genes are slightly misaligned and crossover takes place with a break point between the two genes, one chromosome will lose a gene and the other gain one. A man who inherits an X chromosome that lacks a photopigment gene will be a dichromat. If the break point is within the gene a hybrid is formed, which combines regions of the long- and middle-wavelength genes into a single gene. The hybrid may be red–green or green–red with the larger gene fragment dominating the spectral sensitivity of the resulting photopigment. A man who inherits a hybrid gene will be an anomalous trichromat.

Amino acid changes at three of the possible 15 sites have been found to have the greatest influence on the resulting photopigment. Two of these, at sites 277 and 285 on exon 5, are close together. The third is at position 180 on exon 3. On crossover sites 277 and 285 will normally remain together and the spectral sensitivity of the photopigment will largely depend on whether this fragment is derived from the long- or middle-wavelength genes.

Examination of color vision

Whereas the vast majority of the patients that we examine will display normal color vision a small minority will be classified, under the battery of tests currently used in clinical practice, as color defective. For those with a color deficiency this can have an impact in many aspects of their life, perhaps most notably in the choice of their career. Those with a clearly defined color deficiency will be excluded from occupations that require accurate color perception. For example, it is an obvious safety hazard to have a signalperson with defective color vision in the transport industry. However, people with slight color deficiencies may be accepted for other occupations where it has been established that safety is not compromised.

Many different tests exist to investigate color vision, however, it is rare for a practitioner in general practice to have access to two or more. With the introduction of high-resolution display screens, computer-based clinical testing is an area that will probably address this problem in the near future. Until then it

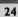
is still commonplace for patients who have been diagnosed with a color deficiency to be referred to a secondary clinic or practitioner where there is access to a battery of tests in order to quantify and grade the severity of the color vision defect.

The gold-standard test for red–green color deficiency, the Nagel anomaloscope is rarely available in general optometric practice as it is no longer manufactured. Tests such as the Ishihara pseudoisochromatic plates, City University (second edition), Farnsworth D15 and the Farnsworth-Munsell 100 hue that are more commonly used, have been audited against this instrument. Although other color vision tests are available only the first three outlined above, which are arguably the most common used in clinical practice, will be discussed in this chapter. The reader is directed to texts mentioned in the further reading section of this chapter for reviews of the other tests.

The Ishihara pseudoisochromatic plates

This is arguably the most common color vision-screening test used in clinical practice. It was first introduced in 1907 and has since gained worldwide acceptance. There are a number of different editions, identified either in numerical order (first 15) or by their year of publication (tests produced after 1962). The full test has 38 plates. There is an 'abridged' version with 24 plates and a concise test with 14 plates. Also a test for 'Unlettered Persons' is available containing shapes and simplified pathways – this is intended for use in infants. The arrangements of the plates are shown in Table 2.4.

Only about 50% of color-deficient individuals can see the hidden plates and so these are often omitted for screening. Transformation plates provide positive and vanishing plates negative evidence of color vision deficiency, with a large percentage of color-deficient people making at least 12 errors on these 16 plates. The test is not intended to grade severity, however, people with very slight color deficiency make less than eight errors.

The serif design of the Ishihara numerals can cause misreading by some color normals who 'fill in' partial loops resulting in for

Table 2.4 **Design and function of the 25 numeric plates of the 38-plate design. Note the remaining 13 are pathways**

Plate(s)	Function	Intended design
1	Introduction	Seen by all, used to demonstrate task and detect malingerers
2–9 Transformation	Screening	The correct number seen by color normals and either a different or no number seen by the red–green deficient
10–17 Vanishing	Screening	A number is seen by the color deficient but not by red–green deficient
18–21	Screening	No number seen by color normals but seen by the red–green deficient
22–25 Classification – only used when screening plates identify a color deficiency	Classification of protan and deutan deficiency	Protans see the number on the right and deutans see the number on the left. If both numbers are seen but screening implies there is a color deficiency the relative contrast of the two numbers will help determine the nature of the defect. The less clear number is assumed to be the one that cannot be seen. People with severe red–green deficiency, especially protanopes, cannot see either classification number

example, 5 becoming 6 or 3 becoming 8. On the vanishing plates, these are not regarded as error and should not be interpreted as a failure. However, completing partial loops on the transformation plates may give an ambiguous result if the reported number is an amalgamation of the correct and transformed numerals. This type of misinterpretation is sometimes referred to as a 'partial error' and can be made by both color normal and the deficient. Color-deficient people however invariably make clear errors on other plates and there is therefore no uncertainty of the overall result. If misreadings and misinterpretations are put into context, 100% specificity and over 90% sensitivity can be achieved.

About 40% of color-deficient people identified by the screening plates are able to see both classification numerals on the protan/deutan classification plates. This result suggests a slight anomalous trichromacy. The correct classification is achieved by asking the subject to compare the clarity of the numerals. The less clear numeral is designated as not seen, thus allowing classification. In more severe color deficiency, usually protanopia, neither classification numeral can be seen.

The correct form of presentation involves showing the plate to the patient for only a few seconds and then requiring them to make an immediate verbal response. Undue hesitation suggests a slight color deficiency. In the 38-plate test, plates 26–38 contain pathways that are intended for the examination of nonverbal patients. Drawing over these pathways takes too long for the design to be effective and so these plates are not recommended. Alternatives include the 'Test for Unlettered Persons' or the Color Vision Testing Made Easy Test (the latter is available only in the US).

The 38-plate test can be shortened using a minimum of six of the most efficient screening plates. The recommended are: four of the transformation plates (plate 2, 3, 5 and 9) and two vanishing plates (plates 12 and 16). The introductory plate and a classification plate should also be included in this approach. A different selection of plates may be better for younger children who interpret low numbers better – plate 1 (introduction), plates 6 and 7 (transformation), plates 10 and 14 (vanishing) and plate 24 (classification).

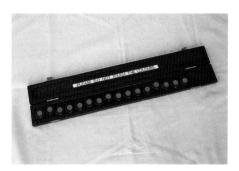

Figure 2.2 The Farnsworth D15 test (reproduced with permission from Doshi & Harvey *Investigative Techniques and Ocular Examination*, Butterworth-Heinemann 2003)

The Farnsworth D15 test

This test, used throughout the world as a grading test for occupation selection, was introduced in 1947. The patient has to arrange 15 moveable hue samples into a natural color sequence, starting from the reference color (see Figure 2.2). The test divides people into two groups. The first is those with normal color vision or a slight deficiency who pass. The second group consists of those with moderate to severe color vision deficiency, who fail the test.

One transposition of adjacent colors is allowed and regarded as a pass. A single error of two or more color steps is a fail. The color arrangement made by a patient is recorded on a circular diagram that represents the hues. Isochromatic color confusions give rise to lines that cross the diagram, showing that colors from opposites sides of the hue circle have been placed next to each other in the arrangement. The color-difference steps are not uniform across the hue circle and isochromatic confusions with smaller steps are made more readily. Two grades of deficiency (moderate and severe) can be identified from the isochromatic confusions made (see Figure 2.3). Desaturated versions of the D15 test are also available for the evaluation of acquired color deficiencies (the Adams and Lanthony tests).

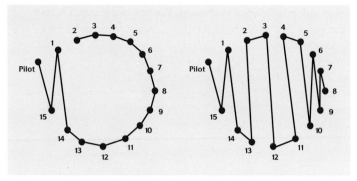

Figure 2.3 Examples of D15 results obtained in moderate and severe protan color deficiency (reproduced with permission from Doshi & Harvey *Investigative Techniques and Ocular Examination*, Butterworth-Heinemann 2003)

The City University test

The first and second editions of the City University tests are derived from the D15 test. These tests have only really gained popularity in the UK. There are ten plates; each displays a central color and four peripheral colors. The patient is asked to select the peripheral color that most looks like the central 'test' color. Three of the four peripheral colors are typical isochromatic confusion colors in protan, deutan and tritan deficiency. The fourth is an adjacent color in the D15 sequence and is the intended choice for a color-normal patient. Like the D15 the City University test identifies only those with a moderate to severe color deficiency. Those with a slight deficiency pass without error.

The second edition has six of the original designs and four that contain desaturated Munsell colors. However, the desaturated designs do not effectively identify people with moderate color deficiency who fail these plates only. A design problem of the City University test results in ambiguous protan/deutan classification in more than 60% of patients who fail the test. However, the majority classification result gives the correct classification in 80% of cases. The number of errors is related to the severity of the

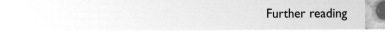
color vision deficiency in deutans, but not in protans. Deutans who make five or more errors have severe color deficiency.

Similar colors are used in the D15 and City University tests, however, the visual task is different. About the same percentage of people fail both tests, but only 60% of those fail both. More protans fail the D15 and more deutans fail the City University test. Despite its limitations the City University (second edition) is useful for identifying moderate and severe color deficiency where a format different to the D15 is required.

The City University test third edition (1998) has different aims and includes entirely new designs intended for color vision screening. The task is to identify colors that look the same or different, and is not used in any other test. The parameters of the test have not been published and there has been no audit of the test performance. Only four of the six grading plates are reproduced from the first two editions.

Further reading

Birch J (2001) Colour Vision Examination. In: Doshi S and Harvey W (eds) *Investigative Techniques and Ocular Examination*, pp 13–24. Butterworth-Heinemann, Optician: Oxford, UK.

Birch J (1997) Efficiency of the Ishihara plates in identifying red-green colour deficiency. *Ophthalm Physiol Optics* **17**: 403–408.

Birch J (1997) Clinical use of the City University (2nd edition). *Ophthalm Physiol Optics* **17**: 466–472.

Neitz J, Neitz M and Kainz PM (1996) Visual pigment gene structure and the severity of human colour vision defects. *Science* **274**: 801–804.

3
Principles of the slit-lamp biomicroscope

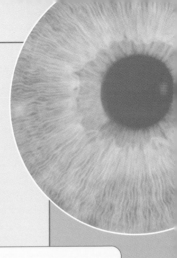

Introduction

The slit-lamp biomicroscope is arguably the most widely used instrument in the ophthalmic profession. Although it is commonly thought of as an instrument for the examination of the anterior segment, with appropriate attachments all ocular structures may be viewed with a slit-lamp. Additionally, with the relevant adaptations the slit-lamp biomicroscope can be utilized to measure a number of ocular parameters, including: corneal thickness and topography, anterior chamber depth, intraocular pressure and corneal sensitivity. With the ease of accessibility to digital imaging, slit-lamp biomicroscopes are at the cornerstone of modern ocular photography (see *Imaging,* in this series, by James Wolfshon). In ophthalmology, the slit-lamp has become the platform for delivery of laser therapy for many ocular disorders.

With its many uses, it is perhaps not surprising that a slit-lamp examination would be high on the order of most practitioners' routine. However, in order to fully utilize the benefits of this instrument it is important that the clinician understands the basic principle of the instrument and its use.

The modern slit-lamp biomicroscope consists of two major components: the observation (a compound binocular microscope) and the illumination systems. The observation systems of most modern instruments have a magnification range between 5 and 40×. Whereas a high magnification would seem desirable, its use often compromises the overall image quality (resolution). The main factor governing the image resolution of a slit-lamp biomicroscope is the numerical aperture (NA). This parameter in turn is governed by four key factors:

- the diameter of the objective lens (the larger the better)
- the working distance (the shorter the better)
- the refractive index between the objective and the eye (the higher the better)
- wavelength of light (the shorter the better).

Optimization of the above parameters to achieve the best possible resolution would seem the best option for maximizing

NA, however, increasing or decreasing these parameters to achieve the best possible result can have negative effects as well. Therefore a balance has to be achieved between NA and the overall image resolution.

The illumination system of a modern slit lamp projects a uniform bright image of a slit onto the plane of focus. The ability of a system to project a very sharp, very thin and undistorted slit is crucial to obtaining a true representation of the ocular structures. Obviously, light used has to be within the visible spectrum. The spectral transmission of the source is also important, the greater the color temperature the better it is to view small particular matter such as debris in the tear film. This is because these structures become visible as a result of scatter, which is inversely related to the wavelength of light. As the structure becomes bigger scatter becomes less dependent on wavelength. Color rendering also has to be optimized in any slit-lamp system as some disease processes lead to subtle color changes that would be missed if color rendering were poor.

Set up

In normal usage the observation and illumination systems have a common focal plane that lies in the same plane as the mechanical pivot of the systems. Prior to using the slit-lamp (on a daily basis) it is generally recommended that the slit-lamp eyepieces are focused. This is achieved by placing a focusing rod in the hole of the central pivot. A focused slit will appear on the rod and the eyepieces are adjusted individually so that the grainy appearance of the rod is clearly visible through each eyepiece. This procedure is performed at high magnification in order to maximize accuracy.

Once both eyepieces have been focused the separation between them is adjusted to allow for comfortable binocular viewing. It is advisable to use the focusing rod as the target. Alternative methods such as focusing on the patient's closed eyelids are often lengthier and fraught with complications and are rarely advised. In a correctly focused and coupled instrument, rotating either of the components of the slit-lamp about the pivot results in neither going out of focus with respect to each other. This means that the angle between the systems (the angle of separation) can be altered without loss of focus (see Figure 3.1).

Examination techniques

Each examination technique is as individual as the practitioner utilizing it. There can be no prescriptive guidelines on the use of this instrument. In the following chapter a general slit-lamp routine will be discussed. However, in the context of this chapter it is helpful to discuss examination in the form of illumination techniques. The five recognized techniques are: diffuse illumination, sclerotic scatter, direct illumination, specular reflection and retro-illumination.

Diffuse illumination

This is generally utilized when an overview of the ocular surface and adnexa is required. A simple way of performing this technique is to use a broad beam and scan across the eye in a zigzag pattern. The angle between the observation and illumination systems is kept relatively wide (>45°) and low magnification is used, to give a good depth of focus. The disadvantage of employing this approach is that it affords the viewer only a sequential view of the eye. A more refined technique is to use a diffuser, which is generally fitted as standard in most modern slit-lamps, and low magnification so that the whole eye and adnexa can be viewed at the same time. Diffuse illumination techniques are useful when a gross overview of the eye is required. More 'advanced' techniques are employed when the eye or adnexa needs to be viewed in detail.

Sclerotic scatter

The basic principle of this illumination technique is total internal reflection of light through the cornea. A narrow beam is focused at the temporal edge of the limbus at an angle of around 45–60° to the corneal apex. The beam is kept 1–2 mm and its height is

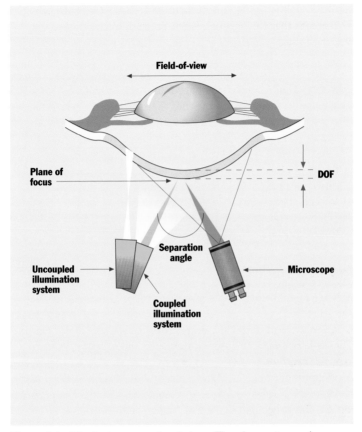

Figure 3.1 The basic set-up of a slit-lamp. The observation and illumination systems are focused at the same point and plane, and the point of focus lies directly above the pivot of the two systems. The shaded illumination system shows how, when the instrument is uncoupled, it can be directed and focused at a different point from the microscope. The figure also illustrates the field-of-view (FOV) – the extent of the eye seen through the microscope – and the depth-of-field (DOF), which indicates the depth over which adequate focus of the viewed structure is possible. Note that the DOF and FOV reduce as the magnification is increased (after Chauhan, K. Reproduced with permission from Doshi & Harvey *Investigative Techniques and Ocular Examination*, Butterworth-Heinemann 2003)

kept between 4–6 mm to avoid producing glare off the sclera.
As the light enters through the limbal junction total internal
reflection occurs within the cornea and emerges at the opposite
limbal junction.

The resultant image produced by the total internal reflection
resembles a halo around the cornea. If there is a change in the
local refractive index of the cornea light is scattered from this
region. This scatter will cause the image to appear bright against
a relatively dull background. Some authorities advocate viewing
sclerotic scatter with the naked eye from the side, rather than
using the microscope, as looking through the microscope could
result in the viewer looking at the apex of the cornea, while
its focus lies in the plane of the limbus. However, at low
magnification it can be argued that the depth of focus should
be low enough to allow both areas to be viewed. If higher
magnification is required in this technique then uncoupling of
the instrument will be required.

Direct illumination

As its name implies this technique allows the clinician to
illuminate the object of interest with the slit-beam and observe
it under magnification with the observation system. A
complementary adjunct of this technique is indirect illumination.
More often than not the practitioner utilizes these techniques in
tandem without being aware of it. With the former high-contrast
objects are readily visible and with the latter low-contrast entities
are often visible. Therefore, using this technique corneal sections,
for example, are readily visible with direct illumination, but scars
may be more easily viewed with indirect illumination, assuming
that the field of view is large enough.

Corneal and lens sections are best viewed with direct focal
illumination (Figure 3.2). A thin slit of light (1–2 mm width) is
directed at an angle (greater for the cornea, less for the lens)
through the cornea. The different refractive indices of the corneal
layers scatter light in different magnitudes and the resultant image
is viewed through the observation system as a corneal section. A
lens section is viewed under similar principles. The clarity of the

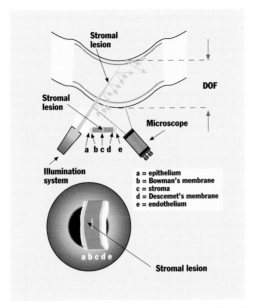

Figure 3.2 Formation of a corneal section (after Chauhan, K. Reproduced with permission from Doshi & Harvey *Investigative Techniques and Ocular Examination*, Butterworth-Heinemann 2003)

image is largely governed by the width of the slit, with a sharper image being obtained with a narrower beam. Reduction of the slit width usually results in a reduction in the brightness of the section hence the clinician may need to increase the brightness of the bulb in order to view the section with comfort.

Whereas the three main layers of the cornea may be visible in section at high magnification, slight focusing movements may be required to view the respective layers. However, with the lens it is unlikely that all the layers will ever be visible. In order to maximize the area viewed the separation angle needs to be kept small and low magnification would give a better field of view. The height of the beam is normally restricted to the height of the pupil to allow the maximum amount of light to enter through to the lens (avoiding pupil constriction) and fine focusing movements will allow the different layers of the lens section to be viewed. As the lens is viewed from its anterior to posterior surface the angle of separation is reduced accordingly.

It is sometimes desirable to gain a 3D view of the cornea (or lens, although less useful). It is particularly useful when scanning the cornea or lens. This is achieved by widening the beam width once a good section has been obtained. Whereas this results in a loss of clarity of the layers, the resultant parallelopiped allows the clinician to form an opinion about the depth of any interesting feature. By then narrowing the beam the observer can then make a more accurate assessment of the depth.

Conical beam and section

This useful adjunct of direct illumination is used to check for flare that may be associated with an anterior uveitis. It is not too dissimilar to forming a section but broader and shorter. When the ambient light is as low as possible the cone of light is directed into the anterior segment. A bright reflex is seen off the corneal surface and a less bright one off the lens surface. If a continuous beam is seen this suggests flare; sparkling particles within the beam represent inflammatory cells that may be counted. The scatter caused by the particles is known as Tyndall's phenomena (see page 67).

A circular aperture is preferred to perform this technique. The beam is focused in the anterior chamber, which means that in a coupled instrument the microscope should also focus on the same plane. If the magnification is kept low enough the entire anterior chamber should be in focus.

Specular reflection

When a corneal section is formed on the same side as the illuminating system a bright reflex is often visible through the observation system. This can often be a hindrance as it tends to be superimposed upon the corneal section. What the clinician is observing are in fact the first and second Purkinje images. The image on the epithelial side tends to be brighter and is a direct reflection of the bright white light of the bulb, whereas the image on the endothelial side tends to be a less-bright golden color.

Due to the positioning of the illumination system the images are only visible through one of the eyepieces of the observation system.

Specular reflection is the preferred choice of illumination for observing the corneal endothelium. In order to achieve a good view the slit beam is normally shortened and widened. To achieve the best view of the endothelium high magnification should be used, typically in the order of 40× (Figure 3.3). At such a high magnification slight adjustments to the focusing of the instrument are required. Additionally slight adjustment of the illuminating system may also be required to optimize the image.

Surfaces such as the corneal endothelium are visible by specular reflection as they are not perfectly smooth. Light is reflected at various angles, which allows the 'roughness' of the surface to be assessed. Light that is not reflected back towards the microscope appears dark whereas that which is reflected back appears light.

Retro-illumination

Viewing certain ocular structures with direct illumination sometimes poses difficulty, either as a result of their proximity or as a result of their structure. Take for example the limbal vasculature, its close proximity to the corneo–scleral junction often results in excessive glare from the sclera when viewed in direct illumination (Figure 3.4). Indirect illumination is often more beneficial, however the relative lack of illumination often makes these fine vessels difficult to see. Another example is corneal nerves, which are notoriously difficult to see as they enter the cornea beyond the limbus. In both examples these structures are best viewed by illuminating them from behind rather than directly in front.

As the name indicates retro-illumination involves illuminating the object of interest from behind. The reflective nature of some of the ocular structures is utilized to create a secondary diffuse source of illumination from within the eye. A good example of diffuse illumination that most practitioners have experienced is the

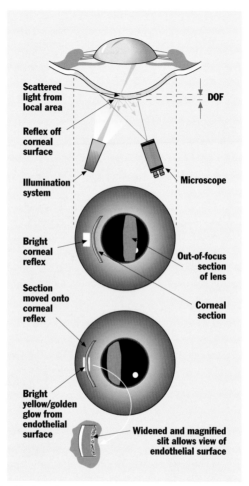

Figure 3.3 Method for obtaining specular reflection of the endothelium (after Chauhan, K. Reproduced with permission from Doshi & Harvey *Investigative Techniques and Ocular Examination*, Butterworth-Heinemann 2003)

dark appearance of a cataract seen against the red-reflex generated by a retinoscope. In a slit-lamp examination the diffuse reflector is often the iris. It is a popular misconception that when

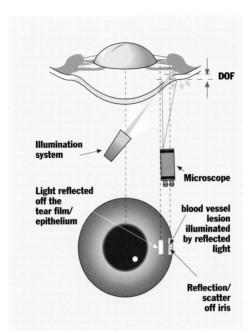

Figure 3.4 Retro-illumination to view corneal vasculature near the limbus. In this area, uncoupling of the limbus is not necessary (after Chauhan, K. Reproduced with permission from Doshi & Harvey *Investigative Techniques and Ocular Examination*, Butterworth-Heinemann 2003)

performing retro-illumination the slit-lamp has to be decoupled. It is only necessary when the corneal apex is being viewed (Figure 3.5b), the separation angle is too large, high magnification is used and the beam is narrow. For small separation angles and areas close to the limbus the cornea (or associated structures) can be viewed without uncoupling (see Figure 3.5a).

Summary

The methods described within this chapter are only to be used as an indicator. It is essential for each clinician to develop their own

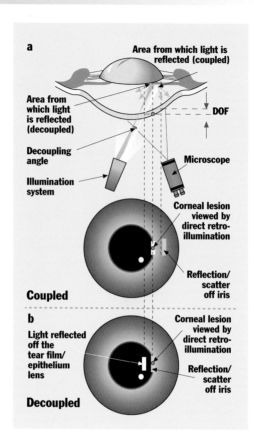

Figure 3.5 Retro-illumination to view an object away from the limbal area of the cornea (after Chauhan, K. Reproduced with permission from Doshi & Harvey *Investigative Techniques and Ocular Examination*, Butterworth-Heinemann 2003)

routine, which should be methodical and effective. Slit-lamp examination is a dynamic technique, with more than one form of illumination technique being utilized at any point in time while the practitioner is making his/her assessment. In the following chapter the application of a slit-lamp routine is discussed to more specific clinical conditions.

Further reading

Chauhan K (2003) Principles of the slit lamp biomicroscope. In Doshi S and
    Harvey W (eds) *Investigative Techniques and Ocular Examination*, pp 27–32. Eds
    Butterworth-Heinemann, Optician: Oxford, UK.
Morris J and Stone J (1997) *The Slit Lamp Biomicroscope in Optometric Practice*.
    AOP/Optometry Today: Fleet, UK.

4
Slit-lamp examination of the anterior segment

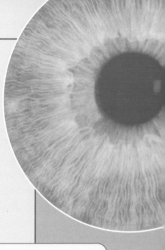

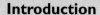
Introduction

No slit-lamp routine can be prescriptive and moreover it must be flexible enough to address a patient's specific symptoms or history. Indeed each examination will generally differ from the last. Thankfully the slit-lamp is such a versatile instrument that it is able in most instances to meet such high demands. In Chapter 3 specific illumination techniques were described to aid and optimize examination. While this is a common way to describe the slit-lamp technique the reader should remember that this could lead to a rigid, nonflexible approach to examination. Moreover, it is likely that in a methodical, structured examination more than one illumination technique will be utilized in unison.

Irrespective of design of instrument the basic slit produced by the illumination system can be manipulated to facilitate examination in a number of ways. These include:

- Slit width. This can be varied between zero and 12–14 mm in most instruments. This can be particularly useful if it is necessary to measure the width of a lesion.
- Slit height. This is varied via a series of stops or in some instruments may be continuous, again this is useful when measuring and monitoring the size of a lesion.
- Slit orientation. The slit can be made to rotate through 180° in most modern instruments. This is usually achieved by rotating a turret within the illumination system. This is particularly useful when fitting toric soft contact lenses where the position of the axis maker can be determined via a scale either on the slit-lamp illumination system or on one of the eyepieces.
- Slit decoupling. Normally the focal point of the slit produced by the illumination system and the focal point of the observation system are at the same point. The ability to decouple the two systems (move the illumination systems focal point) is essential to some of the illumination techniques previously described. In many of the Haag–Streit types of instrument the beam can be decoupled vertically as well as

horizontally, which can be useful for advanced clinical techniques such as gonioscopy or indirect ophthalmoscopy.

The normal white emission of the slit-lamp can be modified with the introduction of filters in the path of the beam. When used appropriately these can enhance the image under observation thus facilitating examinations. The normal filters incorporated in an illumination system are:

- Diffusing filter. These disperse light over a wide area allowing the observer to illuminate a wide width of the object under investigation. When used in conjunction with low magnification it is particularly useful in giving a good overview of the eye and adnexa (Figure 4.1). Diffusing filters come in many types ranging from flip-over ground glass or plastic screens through to a ground flip side to the main slit mirror.
- Cobalt blue filter. This works by altering the emitted light so that the resultant beam is blue. It is most commonly used in

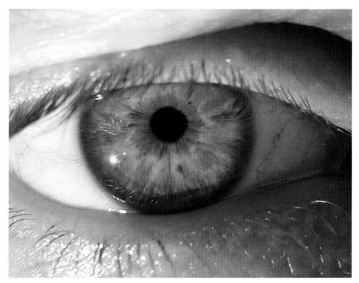

Figure 4.1 An overview of the eye and adnexa

conjunction with a fluorescein stain and particularly in contact lens work, where a yellow Wrattan No. 12 filter may also be used to enhance areas of staining. Cobalt-blue filters are often useful in improving contrast to visualize intra- or sub-epithelial corneal lesions such as whorl-like lesions seen in amiodrone keratopathy.

- Red-free filter. This filter results in the emitted beam being green. The result is that red objects are enhanced, appearing a much darker color (refer to example given in Figure 4.2). As a result these filters are frequently used to enhance blood vessels, particularly the limbal arcades (loops) or new vessels that are often very difficult to see particularly when these fine-caliber vessels are devoid of blood.
- Heat-reducing filters. These absorb light at the red end of the spectrum that are capable of causing thermal damage. They are particularly useful for long examinations as they enhance patient comfort.

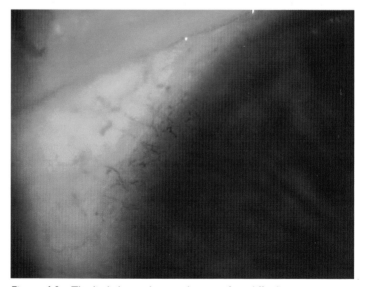

Figure 4.2 The limbal vascular arcades are often difficult to see in white light and can be enhanced with a red-free filter

- Neutral density filters. These have largely been replaced in modern instruments by a rheostat control. These filters are a very crude way of controlling the amount of ambient illumination.
- Polarizing filters. These can be used to reduce the amount of glare and can be useful in techniques such as specular reflection.

General examination of the eye

In the absence of any specific symptoms the slit-lamp examination of the eye can be thought of, in the broadest terms, as a two-step procedure. The routine begins with a generalized examination of the eye and then continues using advanced examination techniques, for a more detailed examination of the ocular structures. Although the slit-lamp is the principal instrument for examination of the eye in a contact lens wearer, for the purpose of this chapter we will assume the eye under observation belongs to a non-lens wearer, although, where particularly relevant, reference will be made to differences between the two types of eye.

In most general examinations it is customary to begin at the front of the eye and move deeper in to examine the finer ocular structures. As such, it is normal to begin with an examination of the eyelids, tear-film and conjunctiva. Observing these structures is generally best performed using diffuse and direct illumination together with low magnification, but if an object of particular interest is seen, then higher magnification is frequently utilized.

Examination of the eyelids

A large angle between the illumination and observation systems and diffuse illumination together with low magnification offer the best set-up for a general examination of the surface of the eyelid. This allows the clinician to assess the eyelid position, examine for ptosis and check for any lid lumps or bumps. The external lid surface should be readily visible using this method and the practitioner should be investigating any localized or general

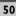
lesions. At low magnification, blink pattern should be readily assessable and this may give the practitioner clues about symptoms relating to dry eye either in contact lens wear or otherwise. When moving across the eyelids the practitioner may utilize a 'Z' or zigzag pattern to examine their surface; moving from one lid to the other (upper to lower or vice versa).

By switching to direct illumination with a more focused beam and higher magnification (10–16×), the practitioner should then assess the lid margin, looking for signs of blepharitis. This tends to appear as either an anterior or posterior form. The latter is more commonly known as a meibomian gland dysfunction. Anterior blepharitis may be either Staphylococcal or seborrhoeic in origin.

Staphylococcal blepharitis typically affects patients with atopic eczema and is more common in females and younger patients. The lid margins are hyperemic and show telangiectasis. There may also be scaling, which forms collarettes around the base of the eyelashes. Where these have been removed, small, bleeding ulcers may be present. This form of blepharitis is caused by bacterial infection of the base of the eyelashes and may be a relative contraindication to contact lens fitting.

A number of complications associated with Staphylococcal blepharitis may be noticed including whitening or complete loss of lashes, trichiasis or scarring of the lid margin. If the infection spreads then styes may result. Internal hordeola appear when the infection spreads to the meibomian glands. All of these lesions are visible using diffuse and direct illumination techniques. The exotoxins produced by the bacteria may disrupt the tear film integrity and also irritate the palpebral/tarsal conjunctiva resulting in hyperemia. Marginal corneal infiltrates may also be apparent which over the long term can lead to pannus and scarring. Management of the condition usually involves performing a strict lid hygiene regimen. Occasionally, in more severely inflamed eyes, referral to a general practitioner for antibiotic/anti-inflammatory drop combination such as Tobradex, may be necessary.

The seborrhoeic variety tends to be associated with a with seborrhoeic dermatitis, which usually affects the scalp, face and chest. The symptoms are not as marked as the staphylococcal form, the hyperemia and telangiectasis are milder and the scales are often greasy but do not lead to bleeding when removed. There are dry or greasy forms. Management involves good lid hygiene and lid scrubs with a degreasing agent, such as an aqueous solution of sodium bicarbonate.

Posterior blepharitis is arguably the less severe of the two forms. It can be subdivided into meibomian seborrhoea and meibomianitis. Meibomian seborrhoea causes hypersecretion from dilated meibomian glands. The lid margins may show small oily globules or waxy collections. The tear film may show excessive debris (Figure 4.3), usually oily and there may be a foamy/frothy discharge along the lid margins or in the canthal areas. Expressing the meibomian glands results in excessive matter being discharged into the tear film. As this is different to the composition of the normal secretions of the meibomian glands, mild irritation of the conjunctiva often occurs. The patient typically complains of a burning sensation, as the secretion affects the normal stability of the tear film.

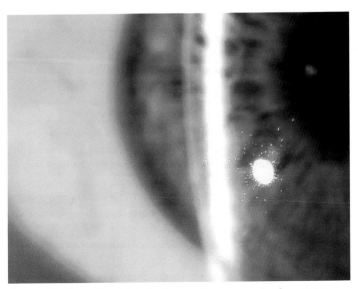

Figure 4.3 Excessive debris in the tear film as a result of posterior blepharitis

Meibomianitis involves inflammation at the gland orifices. The openings may become irregular and are often capped by an oily/waxy matter. Expression of the glands is difficult and any matter expelled may be thick and contain particles, which in some cases resembles toothpaste. If the contents of the glands become trapped, meibomian cysts may form. A papillary conjunctivitis and punctate keratitis may also occur.

With particles being shed into the tear film, its stability is disrupted. Management of the condition involves lid scrubs and possible referral to a general practitioner for oral antibiotics, typically tetracycline-based drugs. Treatment may take anything between 1 and 6 months.

Examination of the tear film

The tear film is arguably the most underexamined ocular structure during a general examination of the ocular surface. Many symptoms of ocular discomfort or asthenopia can be attributed to deficiencies in the tear layer. The tear film is essentially a trilaminar structure consisting of: a mucin layer (closest to the cornea), an aqueous layer and a lipid layer (closest to the surface). Anomaly of any of these layers can result in the patient experiencing symptoms. It is normal for the tear film to be examined following the instillation of sodium fluorescein in blue light (produced by the cobalt blue filter), however, with the reduction in the amount of ambient light produced by this technique some subtle changes to the tear film may be missed.

Diffuse illumination and low magnification offer a good overview of the tear film. This allows the clinician to observe any debris in the layer. Direct illumination or an optical section can then be utilized to investigate detail. Debris in the tear film often appears as particles and can be indicative of blepharitis (see above). The particles are often easily seen with direct (and indirect) illumination as they readily reflect light (Figure 4.4). Large particles often show up well with retro-illumination (Figure 4.5). Particle movement should also be observed. In the normal tear film particles on the surface move slower than deeper ones as a result of surface tension. If the movement of

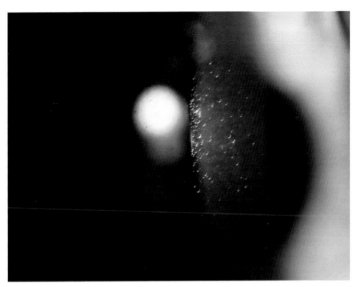

Figure 4.4 The particles in the tear film with direct (and indirect) illumination as they readily reflect light

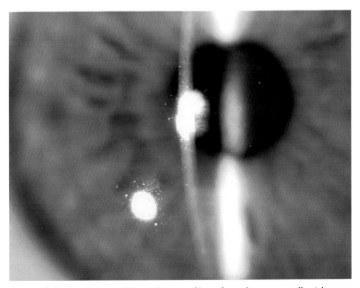

Figure 4.5 Large particles in the tear film often show up well with retro-illumination

particles is too fast, a thin, watery tear film is indicated. Immobile or slowly moving particles indicate excessive viscosity of the tear film. Such a tear film may show interference fringes during specular reflection. As the patient blinks these emerge, like waves, from the lower lid margins.

The tear prism can be seen by direct illumination. This is typically 0.2–0.5 mm high in the center and tapers off to approximately half this height in the periphery. If drainage of the tear film is compromised by a blockage at the puncta or further in the lacrimal drainage system, the tear meniscus height may be significantly greater. This can result in epiphora and may be an important consideration when fitting a patient with a contact lens.

Instilling fluorescein is an invasive method of assessing the tear film. As such there is some alteration to the normal structure of the tear layer. Normally it drains completely from the eye in around 2 minutes. Older patients may take longer as stenosis of the punctae occurs to offset reduced aqueous production. If the drainage of fluorescein takes longer, or if there is significant difference between the two eyes blockage of the drainage system may be suspected. If this is suspected the puncta should be examined. Irregularity of the puncta can indicate canaliculitis. Management of a blockage of the lacrimal drainage system involves punctual massage in the early stages but may require syringing in the latter stages.

Excessive tearing is a hindrance to the patient and is of course clinically relevant. However, insufficient tears tend to give rise to more symptoms and signs. A depleted tear film may give an indication of a tear layer deficiency. Clinicians regularly determine the tear break-up time (TBUT) once fluorescein has been instilled, a procedure familiar to most readers. The eye is illuminated with a broad beam and the cobalt blue filter is in place. Low magnification is used. The patient is asked to blink normally a few times and then ask not to blink. The time taken for dark spots or streaks to appear is noted. This indicates a break-up of the tear layer. Normally, this would take 15–20 seconds, any figure below 10 seconds is deemed to be abnormal and indicative of a dry eye. Where the same area consistently breaks-up rapidly, there is likely to be a surface irregularity rather than a dry eye.

The clinician should investigate this further using direct illumination, optical section and high magnification.

TBUT can also be measured non-invasively using instruments such as the Tearscope or the mires in a keratometer. Patients with dry eye often have mucus strands/globules and debris in their tear film. This occurs as the mucin layer becomes contaminated with the lipid layer as the tear film breaks up. In severe cases mucin may interact with cellular debris to form filaments, which attach to the epithelial surface and move with every blink. Fluorescein staining may indicate a punctate epitheliopathy.

Examination of the conjunctiva

As with the lids and tear film, the best way to obtain a general view of the conjunctiva is to use diffuse illumination and a low magnification. The conjunctiva represents the first line of defense to a series of pathogens and allergens. Any compromise of this leads to an inflammatory response, which is typically visible as hyperemia. The purpose of the overview is to assess the degree, depth and localization of any excessive redness. Dyes, filters and stains all help in the investigation of any anomaly seen, in addition direct, focal illumination and higher magnification will allow more accurate diagnosis of the problem.

For ease of description between fellow practitioners the conjunctiva can be subdivided into zones. Although useful, a far simpler technique is to indicate any areas of interest on a diagram, particularly as there seems to be a lack of standardization between the various systems that exist. Localization of hyperemia may be a vital clue as to the nature of its cause. For example, a discrete area of dilated blood vessels on the bulbar conjunctiva may indicate a pterygium or phlycten. Interpalpebral hyperemia may indicate dryness or an allergic reaction to an airborne irritant, whereas perilimbal redness may indicate a cornea that is under stress.

The degree of redness can be determined by comparing the clinical observations to a pictorial grading scale or alternatively an intuitive scale as indicated in Table 4.1.

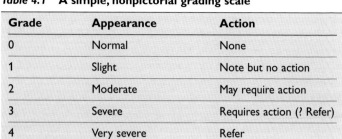

Table 4.1 **A simple, nonpictorial grading scale**

Grade	Appearance	Action
0	Normal	None
1	Slight	Note but no action
2	Moderate	May require action
3	Severe	Requires action (? Refer)
4	Very severe	Refer

If the observations do not quite fit the scale then plus and minus increments can be added to enhance the descriptions.

The vasculature on the ocular surface is best viewed with a red-free filter. It consists of three groups of vessels. These are, in order of increasing depth from the surface: conjunctival, episcleral and scleral. As the vessels move away from the surface they increase in caliber and darkness, with the conjunctival vessels being the smallest and reddest. It is essential to be able to differentiate the depth of any hyperemia in order to distinguish inflammation at each of these levels. This can be done in optical section and moderate magnification by asking the patient to blink. As they do, the superficial conjunctival vessels move, while the deeper episcleral vessels are more resistant. Conjunctivitis tends to produce an intensely red eye and the injection tends to be greatest at the fornices, the vessels which are full of blood appear irregular and can be made to move. They also blanch when mild pressure or topical decongestants are applied. Deeper vessels do not move so readily and do not blanch with slight pressure or decongestants. The hyperemia associated with episcleritis tends to be salmon-pink and usually sectorial. Scleritis produces a purplish hue, which is diffuse and present all the way to the fornices.

Conjunctivitis and episcleritis are relatively superficial inflammations and can either be self-limiting or have some corneal involvement. Scleritis is a deep inflammation and tends to be associated with stromal keratitis and with anterior chamber

(AC) activity. The clinician should be aware and should examine for flare and cells in the AC (see page 70).

A general examination of the conjunctiva is easily performed in a 'Z'-shaped or zigzag pattern. Scanning across in this way will allow superior, middle and inferior zones to be examined. Following examination of the limbal and bulbar conjunctiva, pulling the lids back to expose the palpebral conjunctiva gives the practitioner access to areas that are normally not exposed. It is far too commonly forgotten to evert the upper as well as the lower lid to view the tarsal and forniceal conjunctiva. It is essential to view this area, as this is the regular haunt of concretions and internal hordeola. These rarely cause any symptoms to the patient, but can be the root of ocular discomfort when they break through to the surface.

Everting the eyelids to expose the conjunctiva in this zone is essential if follicles or papillae are suspected. Follicles are lymphatic in origin and as such are avascular (Figure 4.6). With direct, focal illumination and moderate magnification they appear as moderate-sized, multiple, translucent, rice-shaped elevations. As they grow they displace the conjunctival vasculature, hence they appear to have a vascular tunic surrounding their base. They are usually smaller than papillae.

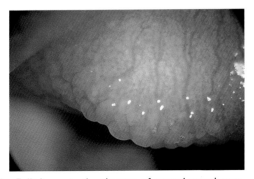

Figure 4.6 Follicles: note the absence of central vasculature (after Franklin, A. Reproduced with permission from Doshi & Harvey *Investigative Techniques and Ocular Examination*, Butterworth-Heinemann 2003)

Papillae have their origin in the conjunctival tissue and consist of a central vacular tuft surrounded by a diffuse infiltrate composed of white blood cells (Figure 4.7). They can only occur when the conjunctival epithelium is attached to the underlying levels by fibrous septa. Giant papillae occur when these septa are ruptured (Figure 4.8). The size of papillae varies greatly, but they are larger on average than follicles.

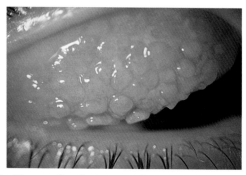

Figure 4.7   Giant papillae showing vascular cores surrounded by infiltrate (after Franklin, A. Reproduced with permission from Doshi & Harvey *Investigative Techniques and Ocular Examination*, Butterworth-Heinemann 2003)

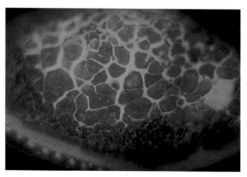

Figure 4.8   Giant papillae: fluorescein makes the outline of the cobblestones much easier to see (after Franklin, A. Reproduced with permission from Doshi & Harvey *Investigative Techniques and Ocular Examination*, Butterworth-Heinemann 2003)

Finding either or both (as they can coexist) does not indicate a firm diagnosis. The presence of either or both is an indication to investigate further. When fluorescein is instilled the surface texture is enhanced as the dye aggregates in the channels between the elevations.

Specific examination of the anterior segment structures

Following a general examination of the ocular surface and adnexa it is desirable to utilize all of the varied illumination techniques to assess some of the finer structures of the anterior segment. These include the cornea, anterior chamber, iris and pupil, lens and the anterior vitreous body. This may be as a part of the routine examination or as a result of specific symptoms reported by the patient.

Examination of the cornea

For the initial examination of the cornea the illumination system should be set at an angle of 45–60° from the observation system and a relatively wide beam should be used in order to create a relatively thick section or parallelopiped (see Figure 4.9). The illumination should come from the same side as the part of the cornea being examined. The clinician then scans across the cornea in a zigzag fashion altering the position of the illumination system ensuring it remains on the side of the area of interest. This method will allow the observer to scan across the cornea in three zones: the superior, middle and lower regions. Using focal, direct (and indirect) illumination allows the clinician to pick up any lesion, which can then be investigated in greater detail using other illumination techniques. Staining the cornea with fluorescein and observing any areas of pooling is also considered an integral part of any routine.

If a lesion is found on the cornea there are a number of factors that need to be determined before the appropriate course of management can be initiated. These include its location, size, density, color and depth.

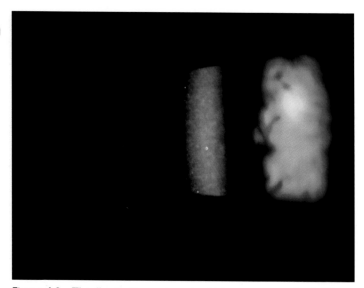

Figure 4.9   The illumination system should be set at an angle of 45° to 60° from the observation system and a relatively wide beam should be used

Location of the lesion

Location is an important feature, which can determine the final course of management. Therefore it is essential to be able to accurately record the location of the lesion. Using fixed landmarks such as the limbal arcades or describing its position in terms of clock face will help the clinician in relocating the lesion and in its management. For example, central corneal infiltrates reflect a serious, potentially sight-threatening lesion that requires urgent attention. Other useful descriptors may be: central or peripheral, superior or inferior, diffuse or discrete.

When a lesion has been located estimation of its distance from the limbus can be tricky, particularly under high magnification. Eyepiece graticules can be useful in this respect; however, many practitioners find the presence of the millimeter scale in their field of view disturbing. The more experienced clinician normally would opt for an estimation based on experience. For the

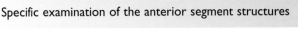
inexperienced comparison to a known dimension, such as the corneal diameter (typically around 12 mm) may prove more accurate. Alternatively, using the height of a beam may prove most advantageous.

Size of the lesion
With a wide beam and low magnification, the size of a lesion can be determined using the height of the beam as a measuring device. Whether the lesion is single or multiple can also be sought. Large, single opacities may be associated with bacterial infection, whereas nonmicrobial agents can cause multiple smaller lesions.

Density of the lesion
Density of a lesion is best determined with direct focal illumination. Most longstanding corneal lesions tend to be dense (Figure 4.10). Some, less dense lesions are difficult to see in direct illumination and are best visualized in either indirect illumination or better still retro-illumination. Decoupling the system and oscillation of the beam to vary the illumination from direct to indirect to retro- may be a good way to achieve this.

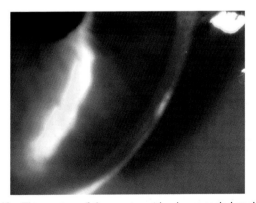

Figure 4.10 This section of the cornea with a beam angled at about 60°, showing an anterior stromal scar, and below it a less dense deeper stromal scar (after Franklin, A. Reproduced with permission from Doshi & Harvey *Investigative Techniques and Ocular Examination*, Butterworth-Heinemann 2003)

Color of the lesion

Most corneal lesions are monochromatic, usually appearing a dull gray. Trauma to new vessels in soft contact lens wearers can lead to the rare occurrence of an intracorneal hemorrhage, which appears red to the observer. Subepithelial iron deposits in the cornea appear a dull brown color.

Depth of the lesion

The best way to observe the depth of a corneal lesion is to observe it in a thin optical section. As discussed in Chapter 3 this is achieved when the angle between the observation and illumination system is large (>60°). Direct focal illumination is used and the beam width is kept as narrow as possible. In a typical corneal section three distinct areas are seen, these are: the epithelium, stroma and endothelium (Figure 4.11). Note that the resolution of a normal slit-lamp biomicroscope is insufficient to see Bowman's layer and Descemet's membrane. The position of a lesion within the section allows the observer to judge its depth.

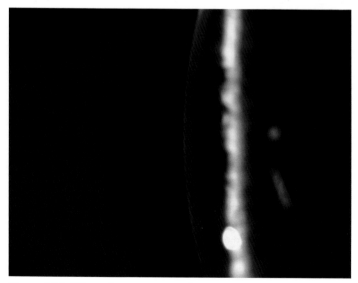

Figure 4.11 Three distinct areas in corneal section: the epithelium, stroma and endothelium

The depth of a corneal lesion tends to reflect the seriousness of its cause. Intraepithelial infiltrates for example, are usually in response to a nonmicrobial trigger such as bacterial exotoxins. Subepithelial or stromal infiltrates are more likely to be as a result of severe infection and often lead to scarring.

In addition to allowing judgment of depth an optical section of the cornea allows the clinician to examine the cornea for any elevations or depressions in an interface. Elevations deviate the beam towards the side that the light beam is coming from, whereas depressions bend it away from the source.

The following three sections are particularly relevant to corneal examination of the contact lens wearer but are deemed essential to a thorough slit-lamp investigation of the cornea.

Corneal vascularization

New vessels are often present in the cornea of longstanding soft contact lens wearers. These are usually most in the upper cornea, under the top lid. To the inexperienced microscopist they can be difficult to distinguish from the normal conjunctival overlay of the cornea that exists in this region. New vessels are generally finer and unlike the normal limbal vascular arcades form tight hairpin loops. They are best visualized with an angled beam and a combination of direct, indirect and retro-illumination. Using a red-free filter may also enhance the vessel appearance. Ghost vessels (or previously perfused new vessels) are best seen with indirect or retro-illumination.

Microcysts

Microcysts are only visible at magnifications of 25× and greater and are only identifiable at magnifications around 40×. They are best examined using a modified technique known as marginal retro-illumination. Light reflected from the iris (and the lens to a lesser extent) illuminates the cornea from behind. Irregularities in the cornea (such as microcysts) can be seen against a bright background of reflected light or against a dark background by looking to the side of the cornea directly (Figure 4.12). By decoupling the beam the interface of the dark and light zones can be seen in the center of the field of view. Under such

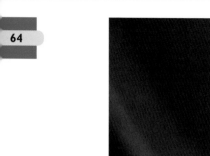

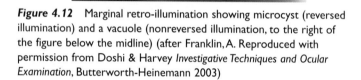

Figure 4.12 Marginal retro-illumination showing microcyst (reversed illumination) and a vacuole (nonreversed illumination, to the right of the figure below the midline) (after Franklin, A. Reproduced with permission from Doshi & Harvey *Investigative Techniques and Ocular Examination*, Butterworth-Heinemann 2003)

circumstances microcysts are seen under high magnification to display reverse illumination. Vacuoles do not display reversed illumination. Reversed illumination indicates that an object has a higher refractive index than its surrounding tissue.

The presence of microcysts is a good indicator of chronic hypoxia and they are therefore most likely to be found where the cornea receives least oxygen. In a hydrogel lens this is likely to be under its thickest part.

Corneal endothelium
Setting the slit-lamp for specular reflection and utilizing the Purkinje images is the best way to view the endothelium. For details on the system set-up refer to Chapter 3. Endothelial cells normally have a flat surface and normally reflect light well, whereas their junctions are poor reflectors. The whole layer normally forms a regular surface (Figure 4.13) but disturbances in size or shape of the cells alter the reflex and produce dark irregularities within it. Blebs, polymegathism and pleomorphism can all produce this effect.

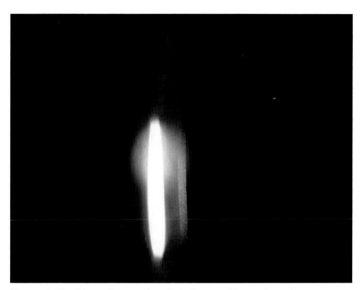

Figure 4.13 Normal corneal endothelium visible to the right seen in specular reflection

Examination of the anterior chamber

There are two principal reasons to examine the anterior chamber:

- to assess for the risk of angle-closure glaucoma
- to assess for any particles.

Assessing the anterior chamber depth

Perhaps the best-known method of assessing the anterior chamber depth is the van Herrick technique. This is discussed in detail in a later chapter. Other methods of assessment of the anterior chamber depth do exist (Smith's method or the adapted Smith's method) but the van Herrick technique gives the practitioner a quick and easy qualitative method for assessing the anterior chamber depth. If performed correctly this technique can be very effective but is not completely without flaw, for example, an anterior chamber can appear shallow using the van Herrick technique, thus leading to suspicions of risk of angle-closure glaucoma, but subsequent gonioscopy could reveal that there is little or no risk at all.

A typical procedure for performing a van Herrick technique is outlined in Chapter 5.

Assessing for particles in the anterior chamber

Non-inflammatory particles

Normally the anterior chamber is largely void of any particles. Occasionally however, the odd white blood cell or pigment granules may be present which are of no significant consequence. The anterior chamber is assessed with a conical beam focused into the anterior chamber. Setting up the instrument for this technique is discussed in Chapter 3.

A relatively common condition whereby particles are readily found in the anterior chamber is pigment dispersion syndrome (PDS). Here pigment granules from the iris are translocated throughout the anterior and posterior chambers. The result is to cause blockage at the anterior chamber, which can lead to glaucoma. Pigment is shed because of rubbing between the lens and the posterior pigment layer of the iris.

The incidence of PDS is stated as being around 2.5% but the risk of glaucoma in PDS can be as high as 50%. The incidence between male and female is similar, but males are five times more likely to develop pigmentary glaucoma. There is also an association with moderate degrees of myopia and lattice degeneration.

There are a triad of diagnostic signs associated with PDS:

- Krukenberg's spindle
- trabecular meshwork pigmentation
- iris transillumination defects.

Krukenberg's spindle represents a collection of pigment cells on the posterior surface of the cornea. It is best visualized with direct illumination and moderate magnification. An aqueous convection current determines the shape of the spindle and it is usually wider at the base compared to its apex (Figure 4.14).

Aggregation of pigment granules may also occur at the trabecular meshwork. Normally this is difficult to see without

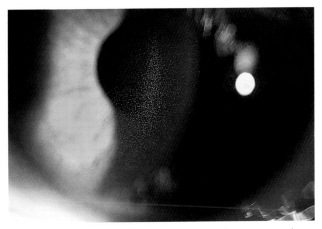

Figure 4.14 Krukenberg spindle in the pigment dispersion syndrome (reproduced with permission from Kanski *Clinical Ophthalmology*, 5th edition, Butterworth-Heinemann 2003)

gonioscopy; however, an accumulation of pigment may be seen on the endothelium at the very edge of the limbus indicating a likely aggregation of pigment at the meshwork.

Iris transillumination is best investigated by illuminating the iris with light reflected off the retina. Light is directed in through the pupil by the illumination system, which is placed directly in front of the microscope. To optimize the amount of light being reflected back the beam height is kept slightly smaller than the pupil diameter. The beam is kept relatively narrow (around 2–4 mm) to avoid pupil constriction. Normally reflected light from the retina in this manner is absorbed by the iris pigment cells but in PDS, where these cells have been shed, iris defects are clearly visible (Figure 4.15).

Inflammatory particles
Deposition of white blood cells and/or proteins is a sign of inflammation of the anterior uvea and may be either chronic or acute. Any detection of such entities without previous diagnosis should be treated with caution and medical opinion should be sought as the underlying cause of the ocular activity may prove to be life threatening.

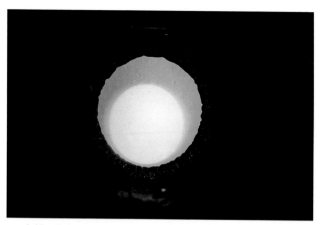

Figure 4.15 Sphincter atrophy seen on transillumination in the pseudoexfoliation syndrome (reproduced with permission from Kanski *Clinical Ophthalmology*, 5th edition, Butterworth-Heinemann 2003)

White blood cells adherent on the corneal endothelium are more commonly known as keratic precipitates (KP). They are normally found in the inferior half of the cornea and often form a spindle shape. However, in acute anterior uveitis the deposition tends to be more diffuse. KPs are best seen with indirect and retro-illumination, however, when they are diffusely dispersed they are also visible with direct illumination. Therefore, the best way to view them is via a parallelopiped that is generated with a relatively narrow beam (2–4 mm), with the illumination set at around 45–60°.

Small and medium sized KP (Figure 4.16) occurs in both acute and chronic nongranulomatous disease. Larger KP, often-termed 'mutton-fat KP' (Figure 4.17) tends to be associated with granulomatous disease. New KP tends to be discrete, round white/yellow in appearance. Aging mutton-fat KP tends to take on a ground-glass appearance. KPs take days to form but can take months to disperse. They may however, persist indefinitely. Older KPs of all types may become pigmented (Figure 4.18). Very fine, pigmented KPs must be differentiated from pigment dusting that

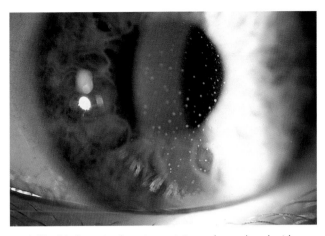

Figure 4.16 Medium-size keratic precipitates (reproduced with permission from Kanski *Clinical Ophthalmology*, 5th edition Butterworth-Heinemann 2003)

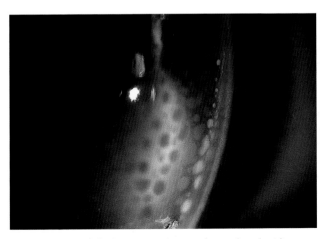

Figure 4.17 Mutton-fat keratic precipitates (reproduced with permission from Kanski *Clinical Ophthalmology*, 5th edition, Butterworth-Heinemann 2003)

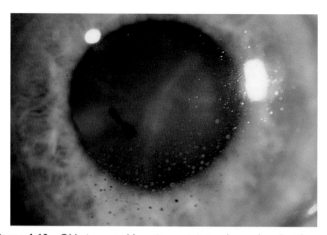

Figure 4.18 Old pigmented keratic precipitates (reproduced with permission from Kanski *Clinical Ophthalmology*, 5th edition, Butterworth-Heinemann 2003)

may be associated with corneal guttatae or pigment dispersion, as the management of all of these conditions is considerably different. An inspection of corneal endothelium, with specular reflection will assist in the differential diagnosis.

Proteins in the anterior chamber, present from dilated or damaged uveal capillaries, cause a relative clouding of the aqueous resulting in the phenomena known as flare (Figure 4.19). Normally flare is present in combination with white blood cells in the anterior chamber but it can persist beyond active inflammation indicating residual vascular damage.

The best way to view flare is via a conic section or a pinpoint beam. These techniques are discussed in Chapter 3. Cells and flare show up in the normally optically empty anterior chamber because of Tyndall's phenomena; the cells and flare are revealed as a result of the scatter they induce. Simple, intuitive grading systems have been suggested for assessing flare and cells, although apparently desirable, in practice these seem to be of little use as the effect is usually either very mild (⩽grade 2) or very marked (⩾grade 3).

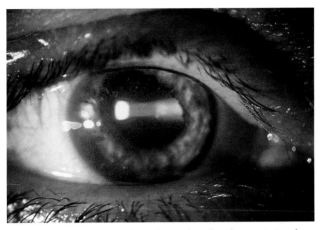

Figure 4.19   Dense aqueous flare (reproduced with permission from Kanski *Clinical Ophthalmology*, 5th edition, Butterworth-Heinemann 2003)

Examination of the iris and pupil

For the inexperienced clinician the iris is a fascinating area to observe with a slit-lamp biomicroscope. The crypts, pigment ruff and vasculature are all readily visible with direct, focal illumination, with the angle of illumination set between 20° and 30° and a moderate beam width and magnification.

In a patient presenting with symptoms or a history indicative of anterior uveitis the routine (and perhaps cursory) investigation of the iris surface needs to be refined. Granulomatous disease results in iris nodules (or granulomas) appearing on the surface of the iris. These aggregations of white blood cells, which become pigmented over time, are readily seen in direct illumination. When they are located on the iris surface they are known as Busacca nodules, however, they more commonly appear on the pupil margin, here they are termed Koeppe nodules. Their presence is indicative of an increased risk of anterior or posterior synechiae. Posterior synechiae may cause the iris and the pupil to acquire an unusual shape (Figure 4.20). If the adhesions become advanced the pupil may become fixed and bow forward, increasing the risk of secondary glaucoma.

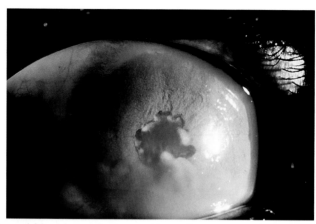

Figure 4.20   Iris nodules in sarcoid granulomatous anterior uveitis, resulting in an irregular pupil (reproduced with permission from Kanski *Clinical Ophthalmology*, 5th edition, Butterworth-Heinemann 2003)

If the synechiae break away following treatment pigment is often left deposited on the lens anterior surface, and this sometimes resembles epicapsular scars. Whereas, the latter is innocuous the former should always be treated with suspicion in a white, uninflamed eye, as it is a sign of previous anterior uveal inflammation.

Freckles are a common feature of many irides. They tend to be benign and remain static. However, a single large naevus should be monitored carefully. It is essential to monitor any change in such a structure. Increasing density, change in color and increase in size all may point to a benign lesion becoming malignant. Slit-lamp-based photography represents the best method to monitor such lesions, however, in the absence of such equipment the size of the lesion can be recorded by using the slit height and width as recording devices.

Iris melanomas are for the most part slowly growing and are three times more common in blue/gray compared to brown iridies (Figure 4.21). They are usually seen in the lower half of the iris and may be either pigmented or nonpigmented (amelanotic).

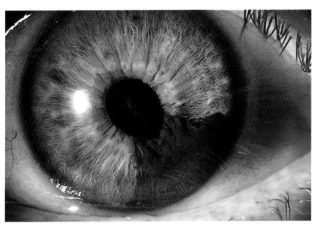

Figure 4.21 Iris melanoma causing distortion of the pupil, ectropion uveae and a localized lens opacity (reproduced with permission from Kanski *Clinical Ophthalmology*, 5th edition, Butterworth-Heinemann 2003)

A lesion increasing in size, spontaneous hyphema, localized lens opacity or distortion of a once normal pupil margin arouses suspicion.

The slit-lamp is an excellent tool for observing the pupil. Nearly all of the methods of illumination described before allow a view of the pupil, however, arguably the best (in most cases) is direct focal illumination. The normal pupil is readily affected in a number of conditions. The affects of posterior synechiae have already been discussed. During an acute attack of iritis the iris becomes congested and results in the pupil being miosed. A sluggishly reacting, semidilated pupil may be present in cases of angle-closure glaucoma. Any papillary defect should be investigated further in the absence of an obvious cause in order to eliminate neurological defects.

Examination of the lens

The lens is best observed using a combination of direct, focal and retro-illumination. With the former illumination technique (see

Chapter 3 for set-up) a thin parallelopiped or section reveals the multiple layers of the lens, rather like the layers of an onion (Figure 4.22). These are more pronounced in an adult lens compared to that of a young child. The layers are most prominent around the age of 40–45 years. The anterior region of the lens appears gray/blue as the longer wavelengths are scattered selectively. Cortical lens opacities typically appear white. This compares to those which lie in the posterior cortex that appear yellowish as they are tinged by nuclear brunescence.

Capsular opacities may occur at either pole. Anteriorly, they tend to be associated with persistent papillary membranes, whereas posteriorly they tend to be linked to hyaloid membranes. A Mittendorf dot is a discrete, white, round opacity found close to or on the posterior capsule. It is often attached to a hyaloid remnant. Sometimes capsular anomalies are associated with defects of the subjacent cortical fibers. This produces a repeated defect over time.

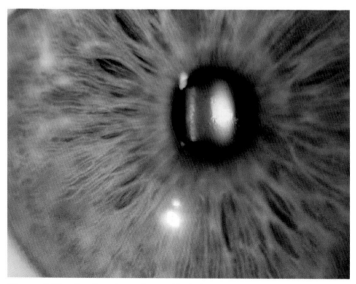

Figure 4.22   Section through an elderly lens produced by direct illumination

Opacities at the posterior pole have more affect on vision compared to anterior defects, because of their closer proximity to the nodal point of the eye. This is also true of subcapsular opacities which may arise from age related changes or inflammation or from degenerative conditions such as retinitis pigmentosa. This effect is most noticeable in bright light when the pupil constricts.

Nuclear cataract can occur in the very young but is most common in the elderly. In the child the defect is initially subcapsular and gradually becomes more central as the child ages, as new fibers are laid down. If the subsequent fibers are normal, an optical section would reveal a lamellar cataract. Nuclear cataract appears yellow/brown in section and they absorb blue light (Figure 4.23).

Retro-illumination used to investigate the lens can also be demonstrated with a retinoscope or an ophthalmoscope. The slit-lamp technique involves the same principle – observing any defect illuminated from behind by light reflected from the retina. The microscope is placed in the straight-ahead position with the lamp

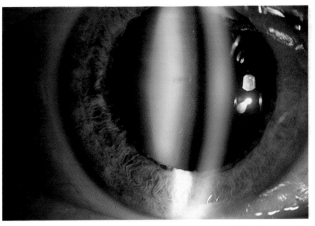

Figure 4.23 Brunescent nuclear cataract (reproduced with permission from Kanski *Clinical Ophthalmology*, 5th edition, Butterworth-Heinemann 2003)

nearly coaxial (but allowing binocular viewing). The microscope is then focused on the object under consideration; the beam is then decoupled and swung so that it enters the pupil near the margin. The beam should be around 4 mm in width and the height is adjusted to avoid any unnecessary reflections from the iris. Retro-illumination is particularly useful in observing cortical cataract (see Figure 4.24), but can also be used to differentiate water clefts from true opacities. Lens vacuoles are also prominent with retro-illumination.

Examination of the anterior vitreous

Examination of the anterior vitreous is difficult as the overlying structures cause scatter thus interfering with the final image produced. Although tricky, examination of the anterior vitreous is important as it can provide useful information about inflammation or retinal detachment in a symptomatic patient.

The part of the vitreous cavity that is normally visible without supplementary lenses is normally acellular. The area that is visible

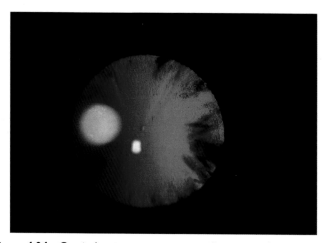

Figure 4.24 Cortical cataract seen on retro-illumination (reproduced with permission from Kanski *Clinical Ophthalmology*, 5th edition, Butterworth-Heinemann 2003)

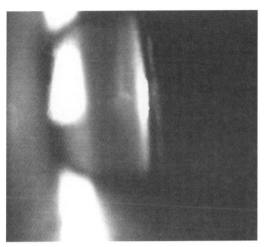

Figure 4.25 Berger's space (after Franklin, A. Reproduced with permission from Doshi & Harvey *Investigative Techniques and Ocular Examination*, Butterworth-Heinemann 2003)

varies with refraction, being most visible in aphakes and high hyperopes. The most anterior structure of the vitreous visible is a thin optically reflective membrane. This is separated from the posterior lens surface by a space known as Berger's space (Figure 4.25). This space is present over the central 8–9 mm, being enclosed by Weiger's ligament, a zone of attachment between the vitreous face and the lens capsule. In pigment dispersion syndrome, pigment may translocate to accumulate at this attachment, giving rise to a ring deposit known as the Scheie line.

The framework of collagen fibers forming the vitreous gel may become more apparent as it becomes less homogeneous with age. The collagen fibers aggregate into coarse bundles and are more visible as they become irregular and tortuous. Any opacification of the vitreous renders this area more easily visible.

White blood cells and/or proteinaceous flare in the vitreous is a sign of intermediate or posterior uveitis. The presence of pigmented cells in Berger's space and the anterior vitreous is a very important sign of a retinal break and often presents in an asymptomatic patient.

Summary

There are a number of pathologies that have been described in this chapter that the practitioner should be aware of during the course of their (routine) slit-lamp investigation. However, this chapter is not an exhaustive list of the maladies that can affect the anterior segment, only some of the more common conditions have been described. It is essential when performing an examination of the anterior segment that the practitioner is only too aware of the potential for pathology to be present.

As indicated before, a slit-lamp examination is a dynamic process, with many forms of investigative illumination techniques being utilized at the same time. Each routine will vary between patients depending on their specific symptoms or history; the slit-lamp is a highly adaptable instrument allowing the routine to be modified as required. It is essential that the clinician is equally adaptable in their approach.

Further reading

Catania LJ (1988) *Primary Care of the Anterior Segment*, 2nd edition. Appleton & Lange: Norwalk, NJ.

Elliott DB (1997) *Clinical Procedures in Primary Eyecare*, pp 177–180. Butterworth-Heinemann: Oxford, UK.

Franklin A (2002) Clinical use of the slit lamp biomicroscope. In: Doshi S and Harvey W (eds) *Investigative Techniques and Ocular Examination*, pp 33–51. Butterworth-Heinemann, Optician. Oxford, UK.

Henson D (1996) Slit lamps. In: Henson D (ed) *Optometric Instrumentation*, Vol 1, pp 138–161. Butterworth-Heinemann; Oxford, UK.

Kanski J (2003) *Clinical Ophthalmology: A Systematic Approach*. Butterworth-Heinemann; Oxford, UK.

5
Examination of the anterior chamber

Introduction

Practitioners regularly dilate pupils in everyday practice and need to take some precaution before undertaking this procedure. As well as a measure of IOP, some assessment of the caliber of the anterior chamber is needed to predict the rare occurrence of angle shutdown upon dilation.

Direct viewing of the anterior chamber angle itself, because of the refraction of light by the cornea, requires the use of a contact gonioscopy lens. With the current concerns regarding repeatable-use contact lenses for clinical assessment, many practitioners who work outside hospital departments prefer to use other methods of anterior chamber assessment. Perhaps the most widely used and best-known technique is that first described by van Herrick, a brief revision of which is outlined here.

The ease with which van Herrick's method may be carried out as part of a routine slit-lamp evaluation has led to its almost universal use. This has, to some extent, overshadowed various other ways to assess anterior chamber depth, some descriptions of which are also given. The patency of the anterior chamber is therefore assessable by several means of differing accuracy and ease of use:

- depth assessment – Smith's, pachymetry, ultrasound, Scheimpflug
- angle estimation – van Herrick's, eclipse method
- angle appearance – gonioscopy, ultrasound.

Each technique has its merits. In a general routine, the van Herrick technique is perhaps the easiest method of assessing the openness or otherwise of the anterior chamber angle. It is essential to do this prior to dilation, but also in patients where there may be assumed some risk of angle closure, such as high hypermetropes. If there is a suspicion of any angle narrowing, such as reported transient prodromal symptoms (haloes around lights, for example), or if there is evidence of the possibility of a secondary open angle episode, such as keratic precipitates, then gonioscopy is recommended.

With both Smith's and, particularly the more commonly used van Herrick, it is important to remember the limitations of the techniques. As the most likely area of the angle to initially shut down is the superior region, all these techniques can reveal are whether there is an unduly shallow chamber or if the mid-peripheral iris is closer to the cornea than is typical. It is perhaps most useful if the following are identified:

- Changes (that is reductions) in the grade or depth over time. A chamber graded with van Herick as 4 a year previous to being graded 3 would be more significant than an angle graded as 2 over many years.
- Large differences in the grading between the two eyes which cannot be explained on high anisometropia.

van Herick's technique

It is important to remember that van Herrick's method is qualitative in that it does not directly measure anterior chamber depth, but gives a grading of the depth, and so allows some prediction of the risk of angle closure. A typical procedure is as follows:

- The slit-lamp magnification should be set at 10–16× to allow an adequate depth of focus.
- With the patient positioned comfortably and staring straight ahead towards the microscope, the illumination system is set at 60° temporal to the patient's eye. The angle is chosen so that the illuminating beam is approximately perpendicular to the limbus and, as the angle is constant whenever the technique is used, this enables consistency of interpretation every time the patient is assessed.
- A section of the cornea as close to the limbus as possible is viewed.
  A comparison is made between the thickness of the cornea and the gap between the back of the cornea and the front of the iris where the beam first touches (Figure 5.1)
- The ratio of these two measurements may be graded and interpreted, as outlined in Table 5.1.

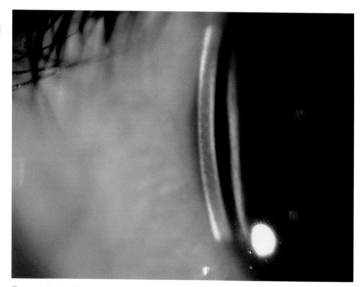

Figure 5.1 A comparison is made between the thickness of the cornea and the gap between the back of the cornea and the front of the iris where the beam first touches

Table 5.1 van Herrick's grading system

Cornea:gap ratio	Grade	Angle
1:1 or greater	4	Open
1:0.5–1.0	3	Open
1:0.25–0.5	2	Narrow, angle closure possible
1:less than 0.25	1	Narrower angle, closure likely
Closed	0	Angle-closure glaucoma
Examination of the anterior chamber of angle and depth.		

- Many authorities recommend a measure at the nasal limbus also, and that if a large variation is found the narrower angle be considered. When the nasal measurement is carried out on many patients, to avoid the patient's nose with the light beam is problematic. Thus, it is often useful to lock the angle between microscope and illumination system at 60°, swing the whole slit-lamp temporally and ask the patient to maintain fixation on the microscope. As the nasal angle is expected to be wider, a narrow nasal angle might be considered as more significant.

- Elderly patients, or those with corneal disease, are often difficult to assess because of the lack of transparency in the peripheral cornea. The temptation is to move the beam further onto clear cornea but, of course, if the assessment is not made at the very limbus, the anterior chamber gap is always wide and hence the grade will always be overestimated. In such cases it is far better to make a judgment in the correct position and then to qualify the reading in the records with a note about the poor image.
- The ratio may be recorded as a decimal, for example a 1:4 gap to corneal thickness ratio might be recorded as 0.25.

Smith's method

First described by Smith in 1979, this technique has been somewhat overlooked, but differs from van Herick's in being quantitative, and so provides the practitioner with an actual measurement (in millimeters) of the anterior chamber depth. The procedure is carried out as follows:

- The microscope is placed in the straight-ahead position in front of the patient, with the illumination placed at 60° temporally. To examine the patient's right eye, the practitioner views through the right eyepiece, and for the left eye through the left eyepiece.
- A beam of moderate thickness (1–2 mm) is orientated horizontally and focused on the cornea. In this position, two horizontal streaks of light are seen, one on the anterior corneal surface and the other on the front surface of the crystalline lens.
- Altering the slit-height adjustment on the instrument is seen as a lengthening or shortening of the two horizontal reflexes.
- Beginning with a short slit, the length is slowly increased to a point at which the ends of the corneal and lenticular reflections appear to meet (Figure 5.2).

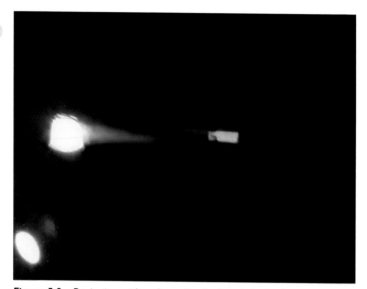

Figure 5.2 Beginning with a short slit, the length is slowly increased to a point at which the ends of the corneal and lenticular reflections appear to meet

- The slit length at this point is then measured (it is assumed that the slit-lamp is calibrated for slit length).
- This length may be multiplied by a constant to yield a figure for the anterior chamber depth (Table 5.2).

Table 5.2 **Conversion of slit length to anterior chamber depth by Smith's method**

Slit length (mm)	Anterior chamber depth (mm)
1.5	2.01
2.0	2.68
2.5	3.35
3.0	4.02
3.5	4.69

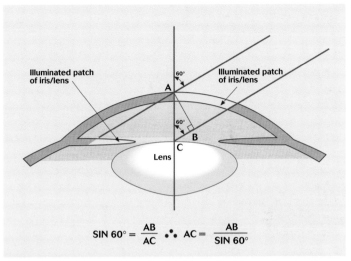

$$\text{SIN } 60° = \frac{AB}{AC} \quad \therefore \quad AC = \frac{AB}{\text{SIN } 60°}$$

Figure 5.3 Theoretical basis for Smith's method (reproduced with permission from Doshi & Harvey *Investigative Techniques and Ocular Examination*, Butterworth-Heinemann 2003)

Figure 5.3 shows how, for an angle of incidence of 60°, simple geometry shows the depth of the anterior chamber can be calculated by the formula:

$$AC = AB/\sin 60°$$

Note that the diagram does not include the change in the incident beam through corneal refraction, and corneal curvature does introduce a variable into the calculation. Studies that compared the anterior chamber depth measured by the pachymeter (see below) with that by the slit-length method showed a constant ratio of 1.4, which approximates well with the reciprocal of sin 60°.

When Smith's method is compared with pachymetry the constant is around 1.31, a little different, but still predicting an accuracy of ±0.33 mm in 95% of the samples assessed. Ultrasonography measurements predict an accuracy of ±0.42 mm in 95% of cases. The constant given by the results using ultrasound, and hence considered to be the more accurate, is that used to calculate the values given in Table 5.2. From a clinical point of view, a chamber depth of 2 mm should be treated with caution when considering pupil dilation.

Adapted Smith's method

An adapted version of the above method has been proposed for use in those situations in which variable slit height is not possible. In this case, the slit length is noted prior to measurement at a point where it corresponds to 2 mm. The instrument is then set up exactly as in the Smith's method, but with the initial angle of incidence at 80°. By gradually closing the angle, the two reflected images on the cornea and lens appear to move closer and the angle at which they first touch is noted. A corresponding value for the chamber depth for differing angles is then calculated as given in Table 5.3.

Table 5.3 **Conversion of slit-to-viewing system angle to anterior chamber depth using an adapted Smith's method**

Angle between slit beam and viewing system (°)	Anterior chamber depth (mm)
35	4.22
40	3.87
45	3.52
50	3.17
55	2.83
60	2.48

Verification of the accuracy of this result with pachymetry results showed a good correlation between the methods.

Pen-torch shadow or eclipse technique

A very simple, though gross technique, involves shining a pen torch temporal to the patient's eye and interpreting the light and shadow across the iris front surface. This may be done as follows:

- The patient should be asked to stare straight forward in mesopic conditions.
- A pen torch is held at 100° temporal to the eye viewed and brought around to 90°, at which point light is seen reflecting from the temporal side of the iris.
- The amount of iris that remains in shadow may then be interpreted as an indication of the depth of chamber. With a very narrow angle, the forward-bulging iris leaves much of the nasal iris in shadow, whereas a deep chamber with a wide angle allows reflection of light from most of the iris (Figure 5.4).

As a very rough guide for use in any situation this technique is claimed by experienced practitioners to be useful.

Biometry and pachymetry

None of the above-mentioned techniques require anything more complex than a slit-lamp or pen torch. However, several other methods of anterior chamber assessment are in common usage, albeit more often in a hospital environment, that require more specialized equipment. Biometry describes the measurement of living structures and, in optometry, is used to described the measurement of axial lengths, anterior chamber depth or corneal thickness. Pachymetry, or 'thickness measurement', describes biometric assessment of corneal thickness or anterior chamber depth.

Ultrasound allows high-frequency sound echoes to be interpreted and provides a very useful method of measuring distances between structures. An A-scan interprets echoes from a single axial beam through the eye, and so gives peak reflections from the intervening structures. A B-scan is the result of a unidirectional (A-scan) beam of sound being transmitted through a medium while being swept rapidly across a plane. The resultant 'fan-shaped' plot gives useful information about structural changes, such as the presence of retinal damage behind a vitreous hemorrhage.

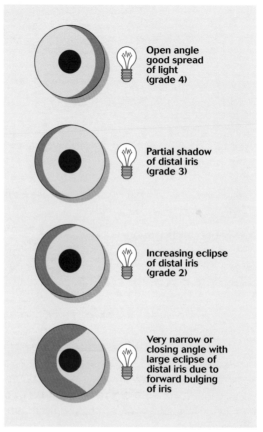

Figure 5.4 Representation of the pen-torch assessment of the anterior angle (reproduced with permission from Doshi & Harvey *Investigative Techniques and Ocular Examination*, Butterworth-Heinemann 2003)

A typical A-scan shows four peaks that correspond to the anterior cornea, anterior lens, posterior lens and retina (Figure 5.5).

A measurement of the distance between these surfaces is therefore possible, knowing the speed of the beam and the time taken for the echo. This measurement of axial length and structural position along the axis is necessary prior to cataract extraction as an algorithm is able to convert the ultrasonography

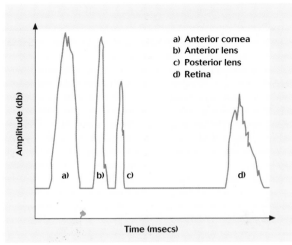

a) Anterior cornea
b) Anterior lens
c) Posterior lens
d) Retina

Figure 5.5   Representation of a typical ultrasound A-scan (reproduced with permission from Doshi & Harvey *Investigative Techniques and Ocular Examination*, Butterworth-Heinemann 2003)

data into a proposed power value for an intraocular lens to be implanted. Many modern ultrasound units used for biometry employ a hand-held ultrasound probe which is held on to anesthetized cornea and several readings then stored such that an accurate averaged reading may be obtained. Central positioning of the probe is essential and many practitioners find that it is easier to do this having first seated the patient at the slit-lamp (Figure 5.6).

As with ophthalmic lasers, the resolution of image and the penetration within the ocular structure of the ultrasound is a function of its frequency and wavelength. Very-low-frequency, large-wavelength ultrasound scans penetrate well, but the definition of the image gained is less than precise (hence the typical grainy appearance of a B-scan in investigating intraocular disease). Very-high-frequency, short-wavelength ultrasound scans have very poor penetration, but the resolution is extremely good. To examine the anterior chamber structure, a poor penetration is of less significance and the image quality is often as good as that gained with light microscopy. Use of a two-dimensional (B-type) scan of

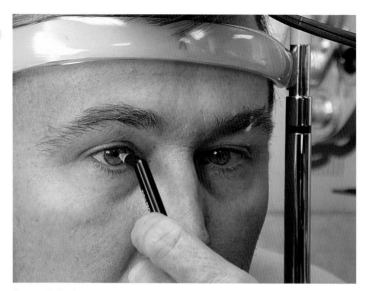

Figure 5.6 Ultrasound A-scan measurement. Note that it is essential the probe is placed centrally.

this nature has been described as ultrasound biomicroscopy, and commercially available instruments have been produced.

Biometry may also be undertaken using light instead of sound. A laser source may be interpreted as to how its passage through the media of the eye alters it. This so-called laser interference biometry has been used (with the Zeiss IOLMaster) to very accurately measure axial length in all but patients with very dense cataracts. It requires an amended algorithm to predict IOL power to the one used with ultrasound methods.

Pachymetry (or 'thickness measurement') is the use of biometry that has been employed in optometry for many years, primarily for the measurement of corneal thickness and anterior chamber depth. Traditionally, the technique was rarely used in general practice and was primarily a hospital or research measurement. The recent involvement of optometrists in refractive surgery programs has increased exposure to various pachymeters. Furthermore, the significant influence of corneal thickness upon tonometry measurements is becoming increasingly important (see Chapter 6). Thicker corneas will result in apparently elevated IOP readings with tonometers (this is clearly demonstrated by the apparent change in measured IOP subsequent to refractive surgery), and there is also evidence that thinner corneas are a risk factor for developing primary open-angle glaucoma. Increasingly, many optometrists involved in glaucoma screening and monitoring, particularly in the USA, are now performing corneal thickness measurement as a standard supplementary test to tonometry.

Perhaps the most familiar pachymetry technique to anyone qualifying before the 1990s is based on an optical measurement. An attachment to the Haag–Streit slit-lamp presents the eyepiece with a split image of a section of the cornea and anterior chamber. Adjustment of a wheel on the instrument allows the back of the upper image (back surface of the cornea) to be aligned with the front of the lower image (either front of the lens or the cornea) and a reading is taken at this position. A correction factor is then needed based upon the measured curvature of the cornea and refractive index to give a depth measurement in millimeters. For monitoring significant corneal disease, this simple technique has proved adequate but for speed, repeatability and accuracy, as well as for measurements mapping thickness differences across the same cornea, the Vernier assessment and wheel calibration is not acceptable.

Rapid, repeatable and accurate measurement of corneal thickness at any position on the cornea usually involves ultrasonographic techniques (though more expensive assessment techniques using a light source may also be used, such as the Orbscan, the Zeiss OCT and, most recently, the Zeiss ACMaster along with various confocal microscopy designs – see Chapter 9).

Ultrasonic pachymeters are similar to the A-scan used in preoperative biometry in that they rely upon a unidirectional high-frequency sound wave, the reflection of which from material interfaces (such as the corneal endothelium and the anterior chamber) may be translated into a thickness measurement. Such a reading requires the ultrasound probe to be positioned in contact with the anterior corneal surface so local anesthesia is necessary.

It is also critical with such accurate instrumentation to note the exact position upon the cornea at which the probe is held as, as is well-known, the corneal thickness increases away from the apex, particularly so superiorly. Also, an artificially high thickness reading may be found if the probe is not positioned exactly perpendicularly to the corneal surface.

Slit-image photography

By directing a slit beam into the eye along the axis and taking a photographic image from an angle to the axis, the depth of anterior chamber may be visualized. By tilting the objective lens or the film plane, it is possible to keep the slit beam in focus as it passes through the anterior chamber (Scheimpflug's principle). More advanced computerized image-capture systems that interpret images from Scheimpflug video systems are becoming increasingly available and should allow storage of accurate information about the integrity of the anterior chamber over a period of time.

Somewhat less specialized and yet more commonly used in general optometric practice, are a whole range of slit-lamp-based camera systems (Figure 5.7).

In effect, the camera allows either digital or analog capture and reproduction of what is seen through the eyepiece of the slit-lamp. In obtaining the best image, the usual rules of slit-lamp biomicroscopy are followed (see Chapter 4), though for maximizing the image captured which is limited often by the sensitivity of the camera system, a few points should be emphasized.

For clear shots anterior to the iris, a backlighter gives an excellent diffuse illumination without causing a localized reflection which detracts from the image (Figure 5.8). For shots of gross external features it is best to keep the slit-lamp beam off to avoid a reduction in quality due to localized reflection (Figure 5.9).

However, any attempt at looking at the retrolental area (Figure 5.10) in an undilated pupil (as one would when looking for Shafer's sign or, as in this case, asteroid hyalosis) proves difficult. The need for a very bright light for the capture is counteracted by the need for a thin beam. Dilation helps, and the slit beam should

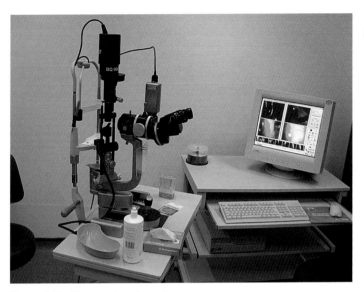

Figure 5.7 Slit-lamp based imaging system

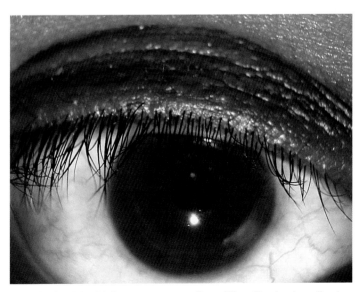

Figure 5.8 A backlighter gives an excellent diffuse illumination, allowing images to be captured of the anterior eye

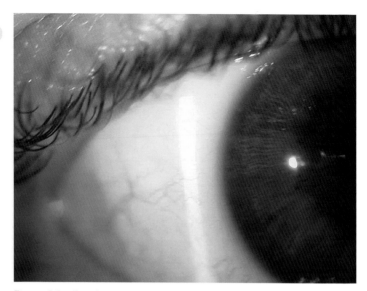

Figure 5.9 For shots of gross external features it is best to keep the slit-lamp beam off to avoid a reduction in quality due to localized reflection

be on maximum brightness and of a height similar to that of the pupil to avoid distracting reflections from the iris.

Gonioscopy

Gonioscopy describes the technique of viewing the anterior chamber angle using a contact lens such that the critical angle of light is changed to allow viewing (a noncontact viewing lens will not allow light from the angle to be seen as the critical angle is exceeded at the cornea and light reflected within the eye). With a gonioscopy lens in position on an eye with an open angle, it is possible to see ten specific structures within the angle;

- cornea
- Schwalbe's line
- Schlemm's canal
- trabecular meshwork

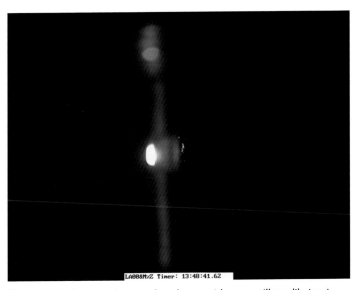

Figure 5.10 Imaging the retrolental area without pupillary dilation is possible

- scleral spur
- ciliary body
- iris processes (not always present)
- iris root
- iris surface
- pupil border.

As a repeatable contact procedure without any disposability development, it is important to be able to justify the use of a gonioscopy lens and to sterilize the lens appropriately between patients to reduce the contentious risk of variant Creutzfeldt–Jakob prion.

The number of structures visible gives a useful indication of the openness of the angle (indicating risk of angle-closure glaucoma), while it is also possible to see anything which may interfere with normal aqueous outflow, such as pigment or inflammatory cells, or neovascular proliferation, and so predict a possible risk of secondary open-angle glaucoma.

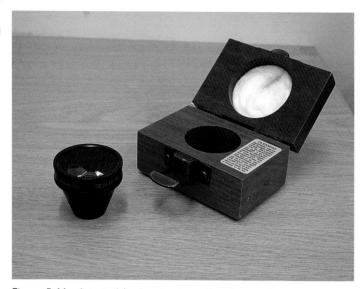

Figure 5.11 A typical fundus viewing and gonioscopy lens

A typical fundus viewing and gonioscopy lens is shown in Figure 5.11.

Further reading

Barrett BT, McGraw PV, Murray LA and Murgatroyd P (1997) Anterior chamber depth measurement in clinical practice. *Optom Vision Sci* **73**: 482–486.

Douthwaite WA and Spence D (1986) Slit lamp measurement of the anterior chamber depth. *Br J Ophthalmol* **70**: 205–208.

Elliott DB (2003) *Clinical Procedures in Primary Eye Care* Butterworth-Heinemann: Oxford, UK.

Pavlin CJ, Harasiewicz P, Sherar MD and Foster FS (1991) Clinical use of ultrasound biomicroscopy. *Ophthalmology* **98**: 287–295.

Smith RJH (1979) A new method of estimating the depth of the anterior chamber. *Br J Ophthalmol* **63**: 215–220.

Storey J (1988) Ultrasonography of the eye. In: Edwards K and Llewellyn R (eds) *Optometry*, pp 342–352. Butterworth-Heinemann: Oxford.

Tromans C (1999) The use of ultrasound in ophthalmology. *CE Optom* **2**: 66–70.

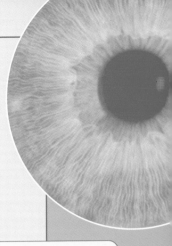

6
Assessment of intraocular pressure

Introduction

The measurement of intraocular pressure (IOP) is an important part of the full eye examination. As well as providing useful baseline data for future examination of a patient's eye, the measurement of intraocular pressure has important implications in screening for eye disease.

There is a well-established association between IOP and primary open-angle glaucoma. Increasing evidence shows how the reduction of elevated intraocular pressure reduces the risk of progression to glaucoma. The insidious nature of the onset of this disease requires that an optometrist, with regular access to routinely examine a patient's apparently healthy eyes, employ a variety of clinical techniques to assess ocular health. The measurement of IOP is one such technique and, as is often the case with a commonly used method, there are many ways to carry it out.

The physiology of intraocular pressure

The pressure within the eyeball is related to the secretion and drainage of aqueous fluid. The regulation of aqueous production and drainage allows control of intraocular pressure, which is important for maintaining the structural integrity of the globe and keeping the refractive elements of the eye in appropriate relative position.

The aqueous is secreted from the epithelial layer of the processes of the ciliary body at a rate of around 2 μl per minute, so allowing complete aqueous renewal every 100 minutes, though this is subject to variation as shall be outlined later.

The method of secretion has been explained to be due to a combination of passive diffusion from the capillaries in the ciliary body, hydrostatic filtration from the blood to the anterior chamber and an active transport mechanism. Most recent research favors the latter of these theories. Passive diffusion appears only to allow for movement of lipid-soluble molecules and the pressure gradient from capillaries to anterior chamber appears too low to suggest a filtration mechanism.

Aqueous passes through the narrow passage between anterior crystalline lens surface and iris into the anterior chamber and drains away via one of two routes. The flow of aqueous towards the drainage routes appears to follow a distinct pattern as illustrated by the way in which pigment is laid down on the corneal endothelial surface in pigment dispersion syndrome (Krukenberg's spindle as in Figure 6.1).

About 80–90% of aqueous drains via the so-called trabecular or conventional route. The fluid passes via the trabecular meshwork into the canal of Schlemm to leave the eye through the aqueous veins into the general venous drainage.

The remaining 10–20% (or higher in nonprimate mammals) passes into the suprachoroidal space from the iris root and anterior ciliary muscle to drain into the scleral vascular system; the so-called uveoscleral or unconventional route.

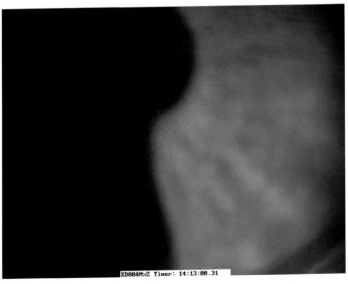

Figure 6.1 Krukenburg's spindle

The range of intraocular pressure in the population

Most population studies among patients over 40 years of age indicate that IOPs measured with a Goldmann tonometer are distributed in a manner similar to a normal distribution with a mean pressure reading of approximately 16 mmHg. However the normal distribution curve is slightly distorted as is indicated by the fact that IOPs over two standard deviations above the mean (that is greater than 21 mmHg) account for 5–6% of the patients rather than the 2.5% predicted by a normal distribution.

A patient with an IOP greater than 21 mmHg on a consistent basis is said to be an ocular hypertensive. The vast majority of ocular hypertensives are detected by optometrists.

For patients under 40 years of age, the IOP distribution tends towards lower values. The aqueous drainage structures become less efficient with age so tending to higher values throughout life, though this is somewhat counteracted by a reduction in aqueous production in older patients.

Because of the dependence of IOP upon the physiological processes outlined, a great variation of inter- and intrapersonal IOPs exists.

Physiological variables of intraocular pressure

There are a great many factors affecting the IOP measurement and which have some bearing on the interpretation of any result gained when measuring the IOP. The following factors affect IOP.

Accommodation

Accommodation has been found to cause a transient initial increase, possibly due to the increased curvature of the crystalline lens surface, followed by a small sustained decrease (4–5 mmHg over 4 minutes measured for a +4.00D change). This

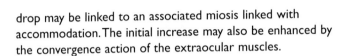

drop may be linked to an associated miosis linked with accommodation. The initial increase may also be enhanced by the convergence action of the extraocular muscles.

Age

As already stated, IOP is found to increase with age, though possibly as little as 1–2 mmHg.

Gender

Females are found to have a very slightly higher IOP (1 mmHg) even when allowing for the age factor in a population; women tend to live longer so are often represented more frequently in population studies relating to glaucoma and IOP.

Genetic factors

Though environmental factors are also to be remembered, the clear variation in IOP profiles between races suggests some genetic influence. In Far Eastern races, there appears to be less of a gender difference and, in Japan, IOP has even been shown to decrease with age. Many studies confirm an increased increment in IOP with age amongst Afro-Caribbeans and a somewhat higher baseline level than Caucasians.

Blinking

It is not surprising that any pressure directly applied to the globe may cause a change in IOP. This is one factor to be considered during many of the methods of tonometry. Lifting a lid inappropriately, or applying a tonometer probe for too long may affect IOP values. A blink may cause a rise of up to 10 mmHg in IOP, a forced blink even higher than this. It is important, therefore, for the practitioner to ensure that, if needing to lift the lid of a nervous patient during tonometry, the lid is pushed against the bony upper orbital ridge and contact with the globe is minimized.

Extraocular muscle action

There is an increase in IOP upon horizontal and downward gaze, the extraocular muscles obviously exerting varying pressure upon the outside of the globe. Convergence may cause an increase in IOP of up to 4 mmHg.

Respiration

IOP increases on expiration and decreases on inspiration. The fluctuation may vary but is occasionally as high as 2–3 mmHg during the breathing cycle.

Ocular pulse

The IOP varies with the cardiac cycle, often as much as 3–5 mmHg between systole and diastole and corresponding to arterial pulse and choroidal filling. This may be due to influence on a hydrostatic secretory mechanism, a direct effect of vessel influence upon the anterior chamber, or, more likely, an effect upon the drainage of aqueous fluid. It is this pulse that is the main cause for the need to repeat readings taken with a noncontact tonometer. A contact tonometer, where the probe is held on the eye for a finite period, may allow a measurement of the IOP fluctuation and some researchers have used measurements of differing ocular pulses between the eyes as evidence of more profound systemic vascular disease, such as carotid artery disease.

Diurnal variation

The IOP varies in a sinusoidal fashion over a 24-hour period, and generally seems to peak in the early morning whilst reaching its lowest value 12 hours later. This diurnal variation may be from 3–6 mmHg as measured in the working day, to as much as 10–16 mmHg if measured over a 24-hour period. It is found that the diurnal range is significantly higher in a patient with primary open-angle glaucoma and a measured change of greater than that expected during the working day (usually 5 mmHg is taken as the cut-off point) is to be treated as suspicious. Conversely, a large diurnal variation in an otherwise apparently healthy patient should be treated as significant. This may be evidence of a lack of homeostatic control of the internal ocular environment and predispose the eye to subsequent glaucomatous damage. The general diurnal pattern mentioned above is not universal and there have been several patterns identified, with some patients having a second late-afternoon peak for example. As well as identifying large diurnal variations, tonometry at several different times of the day may also allow some compensation for the variation allowing one to establish a mean value which may then be compared with the normative value. If, for example, an ophthalmologist needs to decide upon intervention with an ocular hypertensive, they need to be sure that the IOP value they are considering does not merely represent a peak daily value but rather an elevated mean value.

The monitoring of IOP over a period of time, so-called phasing, is a useful technique used in hospital clinics to verify the reliability of a suspect hypertensive referral.

If the pattern of variation between individuals were repeatable then comparison would be simplified by screening everyone at a chosen time in the morning to coincide with the peak reading. Unfortunately this repeatability is not found. This is probably due to the variety of factors thought to contribute to the diurnal fluctuation. Sleep itself would influence the IOP in many ways (dilated pupils, relaxed accommodation, closed lids, supine position, slower heart and respiration rates, absence of external agent intake and so on).

There also appears to be a link with our metabolic body clock that is linked to diurnal cycles of hormones, regulated in part by secretions of adrenocorticotrophic hormone (ACTH). This has been shown to influence secretion of melatonin from the pineal gland which itself has been demonstrated to have an effect upon IOP. The activity of the pineal gland is maximal during rapid eye movement, usually towards the end of a sleep phase, and this is reflected in an IOP rise some 30 minutes later. In most lifestyles this would correspond with an IOP rise in the early to mid-morning.

Seasonal variation

IOP is on average 1 mmHg lower in the summer and the individual variation may be as high as 5 mmHg.

Food and drugs

Though more pharmacological than physiological, it is important to remember the influence of food and drugs on IOP. Water intake increases IOP, as will excessive caffeine. Reports suggest a transient increase with smoking tobacco, but if smoking marijuana or heroin a reduction may result. Many legal drugs have an effect on IOP, such as the well-known link with systemic steroids (increase IOP) or beta-blockers (decrease IOP), but a full list is beyond the scope of this chapter and a pharmacological text should be consulted.

IOP and ocular disease

The measurement of IOP is useful in the investigation of several ocular diseases.

Glaucoma

This term describes a wide range of ocular diseases where there is progressive damage to the optic nerve leading to a loss of visual function and, frequently, a rise in intraocular pressure. With many of the secondary glaucomas and with primary angle-closure glaucoma the rise is very dramatic and produces symptoms, such as corneal edema. With primary open-angle glaucoma, perhaps the disease which optometrists are most likely to be the first to detect, the association with intraocular pressure is not so clear-cut.

Though the very many population studies in this area show some significant variation, overall they show that around 50% of patients developing glaucoma have an IOP of greater than 21 mmHg and that only 10% of ocular hypertensives go on to sustain glaucomatous damage.

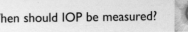

However, before dismissing tonometry completely, it should be remembered that the higher the IOP, the greater the risk of glaucoma. Furthermore, the risk of glaucoma starts to rise above unity at 16 mmHg (not the usually quoted 21 mmHg). Clear evidence for the importance of intraocular pressure in the development of glaucoma is seen in eyes with asymmetric pressures where the eye with the higher pressure is usually the one to deteriorate first.

Therefore, IOP is linked to glaucoma but often contributes at levels no different to that found in the nonglaucomatous population.

Other ocular disorders

As a diagnostic tool for conditions other than the glaucomas, tonometry may often be considered to be of limited use. However, a high IOP reading is often a causative factor in retinal vein occlusion.

Low IOP readings may give an indication that intraocular fluid is being lost. It is commonplace for there to be a reduced IOP subsequent to intraocular surgery and the stabilization of IOP after surgery is often looked for. A choroidal detachment after filtration surgery may result in an unusually low IOP reading.

In eyes with no history of surgery or traumatic penetration, a very low IOP reading can sometimes be an indication of a rhegmatogenous retinal detachment and this measurement may be particularly useful to an optometrist when the tear is in the extreme periphery and difficult to visualize directly. Such a tear has the effect of increasing uveo-scleral drainage via the new communication between aqueous and choroid. A drop in IOP accompanying 'tobacco dust' in the anterior vitreous should warrant urgent action.

When should IOP be measured?

- There are many indications for tonometry to be carried out. Most practitioners, aware of the link with open-angle glaucoma, the major risk factor for which is age, measure IOP routinely on all patients over a certain age. Forty years of age is a cut-off point where epidemiological studies suggest the incidence of glaucoma becomes significant. A total of 1–2.1% of Caucasians and 4.7–8.8% of Afro-Caribbeans over the age of 40 years suffer the disease. The incidence increases dramatically to 3.5% of Caucasians and 12% of Afro-Caribbeans over the age of 70 years. These figures, and the great variability of the disease, are both reflected in the occurrence of open-angle glaucoma in the under 40s, so this author measures IOP on all patients over 30 years of age.

- It is also often useful to have a baseline measurement of IOP on all patients for interpretation of any future readings taken.
- IOP is also routinely measured prior and subsequent to dilation. A rise of more than 5 mmHg which fails to stabilize may be indicative of an induced angle closure requiring medical attention. One should also remember that cycloplegic drugs may interfere with aqueous flow and IOP measurement, even in the very young, may need to be considered.
- Younger patients may present with signs that may indicate a risk of secondary open-angle or primary and secondary closed-angle glaucoma, for example a very narrow angle or the presence of material on the corneal endothelium or in the anterior chamber. An IOP measurement would be useful in these instances.
- Symptoms suggesting possible retinal damage (photopsia, floaters) may prompt tonometry to see if there has been a significant fall in pressure.

Techniques of measuring intraocular pressure

There have been many methods used to measure IOP, some more successfully than others and those that are likely to be used or have been used widely in the past are mentioned below.

Before discussing some mechanical methods available, some mention should be made of digital palpation. Despite this method being largely discounted as inaccurate by many authorities, the palpation of the superior sclera by the forefingers of both hands on the closed eyes is still used, often by practitioners who claim great accuracy. Certainly, a large difference between the eyes should be detectable to an experienced practitioner and there may well be situations, in an emergency for example, where it is the only available technique.

Tonometry relies upon the application of external force causing deformation of the cornea (or the sclera in eyes where this is not possible such as when anesthesia cannot be used and the cornea is grossly scarred) and relating the deformation to the eyes internal pressure. The tonometers may thus be classified according to the deformation produced.

Indentation or impression tonometry

Indentation or impression tonometry rely upon a plunger of variable weight to deform the cornea by a shape resembling a truncated cone. The level of indentation with differing weights is related to the IOP. The prototype and most famous indentation tonometer is the Schiotz.

There has been some renewed interest recently in indentation tonometry. The use of electronic measurement to assess recoil of a magnetically projected probe, so small that no anesthetic is required, is employed in a new instrument (the i-Care tonometer) currently undergoing clinical evaluation.

Applanation tonometry

As suggested by the name, applanation tonometry relies upon the tonometer flattening or applanating an area of cornea. The weight applied may be related to the pressure within and the area applanated by the application of the Imbert–Fick Law (also originally known as the Maklakov–Fick Law).

This law states that an external force (W) against a sphere equals the pressure in the sphere (P1) times the area applanated or flattened by the external force (A).

This physical law assumes that the sphere is perfectly spherical, dry, perfectly flexible and infinitely thin. The cornea fails to satisfy any of these criteria. It is aspheric, wet, and neither perfectly flexible nor infinitely thin. The tear film creates a surface tension which has the effect of drawing the applied weight onto the eye (S), while the lack of corneal flexibility requires an extra force to deform the cornea. Furthermore, as the cornea has a central thickness of around 0.55 mm, the area applanated is larger on the external surface (A) than the internal surface (A$_1$).

To overcome this, the Imbert–Fick Law may be modified to:

$$W + S = P_1 A_1 + B$$

Where B represents the force needed to bend the cornea. When A1 is 7.35 mm^2 then S balances out B and therefore:

$$W = P_1$$

An area of 7.35 mm^2 has a diameter of 3.06 mm and the above canceling out holds true for areas of diameter between 3 and 4 mm; 3.06 mm is useful because if that diameter is chosen then an applied force of 1 g corresponds to an internal pressure of 10 mmHg, so making calibration of any applanating instrument easier. Furthermore, the volume displacement for this applanation is approximately 0.50 mm^3 such that ocular rigidity does not significantly affect the reading. Ocular massaging plays no part in applanation either.

It is increasingly being recognized that the resistance to the deforming force offered by the cornea is strongly associated with the thickness of the cornea. The thicker the cornea, the higher the measured IOP irrespective of its actual value. For this reason, most practitioners requiring accuracy of tonometry also take a pachymetry reading (see Chapter 5).

The very first applanation tonometers employed a fixed weight applied to cause a variable area of applanation, such as the Maklakoff, Tonomat and Glaucotest instruments. These instruments are now rarely used as, with a lower IOP, a force can applanate a larger area so promoting aqueous displacement.

Much more widely used and usually taken as the standard technique is that of Goldmann where there is a variable weight and a fixed (7.35 mm^2) area.

Goldmann contact tonometer

This instrument is widely used and is generally accepted as the international standard by which other instruments are compared and with which the vast majority of research in IOP measurement is carried out.

The applanation is caused by the probe that consists of a cone with a flat end containing two prisms mounted with their apices together. On contact with the cornea, the tear film forms a meniscus around the area of contact and the ring so formed is seen by the practitioner through the probe. The split prism allows the ring to be seen as two semicircles which may be moved in position relative to one another by varying the weight of the probe applied to the cornea (see Figure 6.2).

This use of a vernier reading method adds to the accuracy of the instrument and when the inner edges of the semicircles just touch then the diameter of the applanated is 3.06 mm.

The basic instrument itself, into which the cone is inserted, is basically a lever weight system with an adjustable scale, the scale calibrated in grams to allow varying force to be applied to the cornea by the probe when the wheel is turned (Figure 6.3).

- The basic procedure for Goldmann tonometer use should always involve thorough cleaning of the probe head. As well as the common infective agents one may come across in the tear film, there have been reported cases of hepatitis B and HIV virus

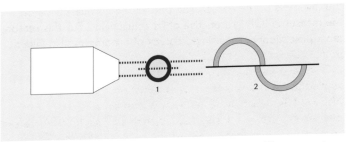

Figure 6.2 (1) Tear meniscus without prismatic effect, (2) tear meniscus seen through prism when the weight applied is at the correct level for IOP measurement

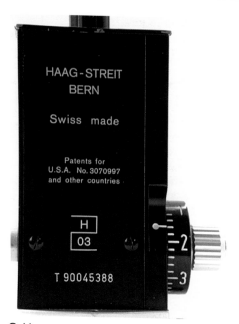

Figure 6.3 Goldman tonometer. Note calibration is in grams

isolated in the tears. The need for disposable contact apparatus in the aftermath of the variant Creutzfeldt–Jakob disease scare has led to most practitioners using a disposable tonometer head (the most common being the Tonosafe shown in Figure 6.4) which is placed within the housing and orientated appropriately.

- Adequate sterilization may be carried out with a weak solution of sodium hypochlorite. Though it is tempting to air dry the probe, dry residue of the cleaning agent has been found to occasionally aggravate the cornea so a rinse with saline is advised.

- The probe should be inserted so that the white marking on the head aligns with that on the instrument to ensure that the split between the rings is horizontal. For astigmatic corneas (of greater than 3.00 DC), it has been shown that the probe should be aligned such that the interprism face is set at 43° to the meridian of the lowest power then the area applanated is

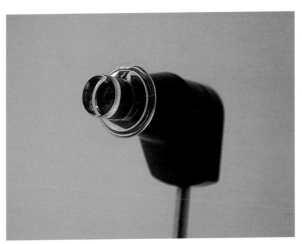

Figure 6.4 Tonosafe disposable tonometer head

still correct. A little red marker on the probe head allows this adjustment for 'with the rule' astigmats.

- The cornea is anesthetized (suggest 0.5% proxymetacaine which should cause less stinging and reactive tearing) and fluorescein instilled. Though difficult to quote an exact amount that would be meaningful in practice, too much fluorescein and therefore wide ring width will tend to give a high reading. If too little is instilled it is difficult to visualize the rings and vernier adjustment is less easy. It may be noted that some experienced clinicians carry out the procedure without any stain at all.

- The instrument is set on the plate on the slit lamp before the eye to be examined and this usually allows the probe to be directed slightly from the nasal aspect to allow the incidence to be on axis despite any slight convergence by the patient. To minimize the contact time with the cornea it is useful to set the instrument to a weight setting of 1 g (10 mmHg) or a previous reading if known. On low to medium magnification, the probe is viewed through the microscope with the cobalt blue light incident on the probe head, the lamp set at 60° temporally.

- The probe is moved on to the cornea and the rings are visualized and adjusted as mentioned. If the semicircles are not of equal size then small vertical adjustments may be needed. If the semicircles are not equal, the reading will be too high.
- The probe should be removed from the cornea, the weight reading on the scale noted (in grams or ×10 for mmHg), and the cornea checked for staining. If staining is induced, most epithelial stain will disappear within a matter of several hours but caution by the optometrist should be exercised; if worried, monitor.

Prolonged contact should be avoided to minimize corneal compromise, but it does allow the practitioner to visualize the ocular pulse, seen as small oscillations of the semicircles relative to each other. Prolonged contact also has the effect of reducing IOP by an ocular massaging process. A reduction in this effect or a marked difference between the ocular pulse in each eye may be indicative of vascular occlusive disease.

The thickness of the cornea may also cause some error as a very thin cornea will produce low IOP readings. A very irregular cornea may make visualization of the rings difficult but a contact method is probably more accurate in this case than a noncontact method. In cases of extreme corneal vulnerability or where anesthesia is not advisable, the contact methods may not be first choice.

As with any accurate measuring instrument, regular calibration is necessary and is easily carried out by the practitioner.

Perkins contact tonometer

The Perkins contact tonometer was developed as a hand-held, and therefore portable, version of the Goldmann. Having its own light source and viewing lens negates the need for the slit-lamp. The probe is held on a counterbalanced mounting with a coiled spring that allows the instrument to be used accurately in either the horizontal or vertical position, useful for the supine patient in a domicilary visit. This mechanism originally required a slightly differently weighted probe to maintain accuracy, denoted by a red ring marking as opposed to the black ring marking on Goldmann

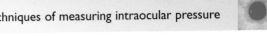

probes. The advent of newer designs of both instrument and probe has done away with this discrepancy.

The instrument has a headrest attachment that may be extended and held in position on the patient's forehead to minimize instrument shake, possibly one of the main problems with this instrument. The Mark II version now available has two light sources for ease of viewing and may be fitted with a magnifying device (the Perkins examination telescope) allowing viewing of the rings at arm's length.

Tonosafe probes may be used with this instrument. Its operation is as with the Goldmann. Calibration should be carried out regularly and may be done by the practitioner.

Not surprisingly, the results gained are comparable to the Goldmann.

Tonopen XL Mentor

The Tonopen XL Mentor is a small, portable electronic contact tonometer which has a stainless steel probe which, on contact with the cornea, measures IOP by an electronic signal from a solid-state strain gauge held within. The short contact time requires several readings to be taken and averaged, but this, combined with its small appearance, appears to make it patient friendly.

Results appear to be reliable in comparison with the Goldmann, albeit with some greater spread as may be expected in any instrument taking a series of instant readings compared with one prolonged reading.

Noncontact tonometers (NCTs)

The NCT was first introduced in 1972 and has the obvious advantage of not requiring contact with the cornea. This minimizes the potential for corneal compromise, negates the need for anesthesia, and in many cases is preferred by the patient. Automation of the mechanism means that the instruments are often used by nonprofessional staff as a screening instrument.

There are a wide variety of instruments on the market, and rarely a year goes by without some new upgrade of an instrument. The basic operation of the instrument relies upon the applanation of an area of cornea by a jet of air which is usually switched on and off at a point dictated by the quality of image of reflected light from a source on the tonometer. The instrument then electronically converts either the time taken to flatten the cornea or the pressure of air needed into a reading of intraocular pressure.

Because the instruments rely upon the flattened cornea acting to reflect incident light into a receiver, anything compromising the reflection (such as heavy scarring or distortion) will impact upon the accuracy of the reading. However, most designs include an 'override' feature allowing a reading to be made even if the received light beam is not maximal. This is also useful if the patient has poor fixation or rapid blinking.

As all the NCTs take an instantaneous reading of IOP, there is some variation between readings. If the reading is taken on the peak of the ocular pulse, respiratory cycle and immediately after a blink then a disproportionately high reading may be found. It is standard practice, therefore, for the NCT to take three or four consistent readings before arriving at a useful value. Most instruments automatically calculate an average. A recent innovation has been to incorporate into the patient's forehead rest a sensor which monitors the patient's pulse. The thinking behind this is to only allow a reading to be taken at a specified point on the cardiac cycle so overcoming any variation due to the ocular pulse. It does not, however, have influence over the other physiological variations mentioned earlier so the days of a 'single puff' NCT are not here yet.

The overall perception of NCTs giving higher readings is likely to be based on practitioners using an inappropriate average or not taking enough readings. In fact any significant studies have suggested if there is any difference it is the NCT being lower than the contact method.

There is now a substantial body of literature comparing results taken from the various NCTs with the Goldmann standard, certainly within the nonhypertensive population. At higher readings, say above 28 mmHg, the correlation breaks down and NCT readings seem less consistent, despite most incorporating adjustments to deal with higher values. It is for this reason, which is becoming increasingly debatable, that many ophthalmologists recommend referral of consistently measured high IOP taken with a contact method, or that high NCT readings be confirmed with a contact method before referral.

There are many NCTs available, a full description of each being outside the scope of this book. Most incorporate a calibration mechanism and a demonstration setting to allow the patient to know what to expect from the 'puff of air'. This action usually also serves to clear any dust particles from the air chamber which could otherwise be transferred to the patient's cornea. Most use a flashing nonaccommodative target to reduce the variation due to accommodation and wandering fixation.

Corneal hysteresis

As already stated, the deformation of the cornea due to an applied force is, to a certain extent, related to the corneal thickness as well as the IOP within. The deformation is visco-elastic rather than truly elastic, meaning that the recovery of the cornea to its original shape when the deforming force is reduced will occur at a different rate to the original deformation. This is measurable if the force to cause applanation is measured and the cornea further deformed to a concave shape before the force is reduced and that at which the applanated position is reached again also measured. The difference between these two forces represents what is known as the corneal hysteresis and may be used to indicate the resistance of the cornea to force and so to adapt a tonometer reading. An instrument, such as the Reichert Ocular Response Analyzer, attempts this and clinical trials will soon show the validity of such a measurement in predicting actual IOP.

Ocular blood flow tonometry

It has already been suggested that there is a close correlation between the IOP and the ocular blood flow. Over recent years a contact tonometer has been developed, the Ocular Blood Flow

Tonometer, which measures IOP, and the ocular pulse in terms of pulse amplitude, pulse volume and pulsatile blood flow. In contact with the eye, the machine samples over 200 readings per second over a period of 7–10 seconds so allowing for several beats of the heart.

As well as providing accurate IOP information, the data regarding hemodynamics provide useful baseline data allowing for interpersonal comparison and changes over time to be analyzed. At present, such measurements are rarely carried out outside specialist clinics.

Analysis of results

It would be a very easy, if possibly boring, world if it were possible to have a list of situations which would warrant referral, including a cut-off IOP measurement. It should now be clear that IOP alone as a predictor of eye disease is not reliable and that referral in the absence of any other risk factor is only agreed to be necessary at consistently very high values.

A safe policy is for the optometrist to find out what local hospital policy is regarding referral on IOP alone. In the practices this author works in, local ophthalmologists are happy to see patients with repeatable IOP readings of over 25 mmHg, and consider treatment if verified to be over 30 mmHg. It is not unheard of for the patients in the 25–30 mmHg group to be checked and discharged with advice to attend regularly at the optometric practice for IOP monitoring. Many surgeons now treat ocular hypertension of 25 mmHg or more with hypotensive agents in the absence of any signs of glaucoma, particularly in high-risk groups such as Afro-Caribbeans. This is in light of the Ocular Hypertension Treatment Studies suggesting such action reduces significantly the risk of any progression in such patients to glaucoma. A very high IOP reading in an asymptomatic eye may occasionally occur in chronic secondary glaucoma conditions, such as Posner–Schlossman syndrome, where the history of inflammatory activity may be vague and the IOP rise only transient.

It is also a significant finding if there is a significant and repeatable difference between the IOPs of each eye (5 mmHg or more), if this finding cannot be related to previous history, such as intraocular surgery, or a significant anisometropia.

As already stated, an unusually low IOP (less than 8 mmHg for example) may be clinically significant.

Further reading

Alward WLM (1994) *Colour Atlas of Gonioscopy*. Wolfe Publishing: London.

Carlson NB, Kurtz D, Heath DA and Hines C (1996) *Clinical Procedures for Ocular Examination*, Second Edition p. 256–263. (Stamford: Appleton and Lange).

Fingeret M, Casser L and Woodcome HT (1990) *Atlas of Primary Eyecare Procedures*, p. 72–84. Appleton and Lange: Norwalk.

Fisch BM (1993) *Gonioscopy and the Glaucomas*. Butterworth-Heinemann: Stoneham.

7
Direct versus indirect ophthalmoscopy

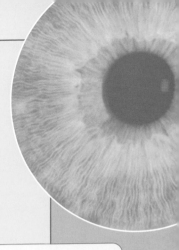

Introduction

A thorough examination of the ocular fundus is mandatory in any eye examination. The routine employed by the practitioner will largely depend on the specific history and symptoms a patient presents with. Factors such as age, systemic medication and race also play an important role and may warrant adaptation to the practitioner's normal routine.

In recent times there has been much discussion about the technique employed to visualize the fundus. The tried and trusted direct ophthalmoscope has come under much criticism, mostly based around its limited field of view. Nonetheless, it still remains the cornerstone of most practitioners' fundus examination routine. With the popularization of comanagement schemes, our use and understanding of the benefits of indirect ophthalmoscopy has grown. Moreover, as practitioners have become more familiar with this method, indirect ophthalmoscopy has found its way into the general routine of many. Both methods have their advantages and disadvantages; indeed many clinicians use both methods to optimize their examination of the fundus. The purpose of this chapter is to discuss examination techniques in both methods and highlight their benefits and pitfalls.

To dilate or not?

There can be no argument that fundus examination is greatly facilitated by dilating the pupil. However, the decision of whether or not to dilate a patient (or indeed every patient) must be based on reasoned clinical decision-making, and not factors such as time or economy. The advantages of an enhanced fundus view must generally outweigh any negative effects of pupillary dilation.

It is still a concern of some practitioners that pupil dilation may induce angle-closure and lead to an attack of glaucoma. Although the roots of this statement are solid, the incidence, which is often quoted around less than 1:100 000, is very small. Indeed, there are experienced practitioners who readily dilate patients, who have never witnessed such an event in their lengthy career. It is important however, not to be frugal with dilation and it is essential that all the risk factors are eliminated before attempting to dilate an individual.

Normal history and symptoms may pinpoint individuals who might have a predisposition to angle closure. Slit-lamp examination may also be useful in identifying patients with iris/angle anomalies who may also be at risk. An assessment of the anterior chamber depth can be obtained using a van Herrick technique (see Chapter 5). However, it is important to bear in mind that a patient with a shallow anterior chamber depth by this technique is not necessarily at risk of closure. The cautious practitioner may also want to determine intraocular pressure (IOP) predilation and repeat this measurement approximately 30 minutes after maximum dilation has been achieved. Any significant rise in IOP (>5 mmHg) may be indicative of angle-closure and would warrant further monitoring. If pressures continue to rise then the local casualty department should be contacted.

In addition to those with shallow angles or risk factors that may precipitate angle closure, it is accepted that there are a number of patients for whom dilation is contraindicated. These are:

- patients with a history of penetrating injury
- patients with iris-clip intraocular lenses.

Driving following pupil dilation is generally contraindicated, however, for patients who need to drive home following an eye examination a supplementary appointment can be made for fundus examination, on a day that they do not have to drive or when they can be accompanied. An exception to this last point is when the patient presents with symptoms indicative of a serious retinal pathology, such as a detachment. Here the patient must be dilated immediately as a thorough examination is required.

There is some debate as to which pharmacological agent should be used to dilate a pupil. The choice of drug may vary with each patient and the nature of the examination to be performed. For example, if fundus examination and a cycloplegic refraction in a young patient are required there is very little point in using a mild miotic drug. Any drop used should be fast acting, able to be effective for the full duration required, minimally toxic, have low risk of any side effects (local or systemic) and have a quick recovery time.

Most authorities advise using either of the following combinations:

- One drop of 2.5% phenylephrine (stimulating the dilatator pupillae of the iris) together with one drop of 0.5% tropicamide (restricts the action of the sphincter pupillae). The synergistic action of these two drugs produces maximal pupil dilation and improves patient comfort as it restricts pupil constriction during examination.
- Two drops of 0.5% tropicamide instilled a minute apart.

The choices above are not prescriptive and the practitioner may modify their choice based on factors such as age of patient, race or patient's general health. It is important to bear in mind that dilation can be facilitated up by instilling one drop of topical anesthetic prior to instillation of the dilating drop(s), as this increases the permeability across the cornea.

Direct ophthalmoscopy

The direct ophthalmoscope still remains the favored instrument of many practitioners. It is probably because of its ease of use and magnified view that this instrument has so long been at the vanguard of fundus examination. As this was the instrument that most practitioners used routinely during their training perhaps this is why it has become an inherent part of most clinicians' armory. The direct ophthalmoscope has many positive features and used in conjunction with an indirect ophthalmoscope, fundus examination can be optimized. Table 7.1 lists some of the major benefits and pitfalls of the direct ophthalmoscope.

The restricted field of view makes the direct ophthalmoscope difficult to use when scanning across the fundus, with only small areas being visible at any one point in time (see Figure 7.1). This

Table 7.1 Features of the direct ophthalmoscope

Advantages	Disadvantages
High magnification (×15)	Magnification varies with the patient's refractive error. Higher in myopes
Relatively good image obtained even through a small pupil	Very low field of view (around 10° in an emmetrope).
Portable	Monocular field of view
Relatively inexpensive	Can be difficult to use on uncooperative patients
View of fundus is the correct way up and nonreversed	Image degrades with media opacities Poor at showing color change or elevation Very close proximity to patient required

becomes particularly relevant when an overall view of the posterior pole is required such as in a diabetic. A small pupil and media opacities further heighten this problem. The difficulties are minimized by dilation. Therefore, for a patient with small pupils and/or media opacities, pupillary dilation is recommended to perform a thorough examination.

The monocular view of the direct ophthalmoscope renders judgment of depth difficult and the observer has to rely on other cues to form an opinion. A useful addition to most modern direct ophthalmoscopes is the inclusion of a slit graticule. This can be projected onto the fundus and any change in its regularity would indicate an area of elevation or depression.

Wide-field direct ophthalmoscopy

Recently launched instruments claim to overcome some of the shortfalls of the direct ophthalmoscope. An example is the PanOptic from Welch Allyn. Using a patented optical system (see

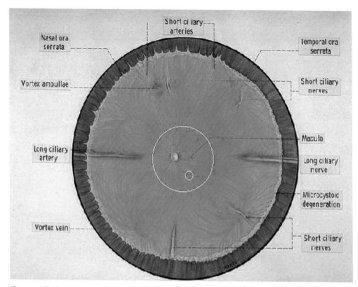

Figure 7.1 View of entire fundus. The larger circle indicates the central area, while the smaller circle is the field of view through a direct ophthalmoscope. Localizing features are shown (reproduced with permission from Doshi & Harvey *Investigative Techniques and Ocular Examination*, Butterworth-Heinemann 2003)

Figure 7.2) such instruments have three main advantages of the conventional direct ophthalmoscope. These are:

- an enhanced field of view in the undilated eye, typically quoted to be in the order of 25°
- a 26% increase in magnification. This results in the image being a quarter bigger than with the standard ophthalmoscope, thus improving resolution of the retina, hence allowing fine detail such as vascular changes to be more easily viewed
- an increase in the working distance between patient and clinician, allowing improved comfort for both.

The optic of such systems differs from the conventional direct ophthalmoscope in that they allow light to converge to a point at

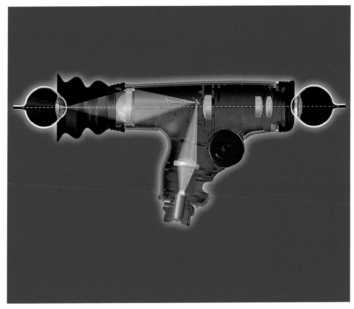

Figure 7.2 Patented optics of the Welch Allyn PanOptic direct ophthalmoscope

the cornea and then diverge towards the retina, allowing for a wider field of view. In a standard ophthalmoscope, light is projected directly onto the observer's retina. The image produced is erect and not inverted. This point convergence makes the distance from the patient a crucial factor in maintaining a good field of view.

Slit-lamp direct ophthalmoscopy

Slit-lamp direct ophthalmoscopy can be performed with a high minus (non-contact) lens, the Hruby lens. The high-powered minus lens (−58.6D) produces a virtual image that is upright and not laterally reversed. The major advantages of utilizing this method are the stereopsis and high magnification can be achieved through the slit-lamp.

Pupil dilation is essential in this technique and maximum dilation must be achieved. Hence an antimuscarinic/

sympathomimetic drug combination must be used. However, even with pupil dilation this method offers the worst field of view of any of the slit-lamp-based techniques currently available. The field of view is typically 20–30° in an emmetropic eye.

At high magnification, any slight movement of the patient's eye or the lens can result in severe degradation of the image. In order to minimize this most Hruby lenses are mounted on a stand (fixed onto the slit-lamp) and the slit-lamp fixation target is employed.

Examination technique

- Maximum pupil dilation is achieved with an antimuscarinic/sympathomimetic drug combination.
- The patient is instructed on the need for maximum compliance and asked to fixate the slit-lamp fixation target.
- The microscope is placed in the straight-ahead position with the lamp coaxial (allowing binocular viewing). The magnification is set to its lowest position and the slit adjusted to a height around 5 mm and width 2 mm.
- The slit is focused in the plane of the patient's pupil. The lens is introduced (concave side closest to the cornea) as close as possible to the patient's eye, without causing any contact or discomfort.
- The slit-lamp is focused by moving it towards the patient.
- The retina appears in view after focusing through the lens and vitreous. Adjustments to the position of the beam and its height are made to optimize the image. The magnification and beam width can also be altered to optimize the image.

The excellent stereopsis produced by this technique (arguably the best of all the noncontact methods) allows subtle changes in retinal thickness to be determined.

Fundus contact lenses

Although there are a number of lenses available on the market, probably the best-known fundus contact lens is the Goldmann three-mirror lens. Fundus contact lenses provide the best degree of stereopsis of all of the methods of examination. Additionally, they allow the observer to view the extreme periphery of the fundus, as well as the central region. It is perhaps fair to say that these lenses haven't really taken off in popularity in general optometric practice, as they are perceived as being difficult to use. Moreover, the need to contact the surface of the eye (albeit with a coupling fluid in place) is off putting to the majority of practitioners.

However, possibly the most significant factor as to why these lenses have now become relatively obsolete is because optical and government agencies have advised against the use of procedures that involve direct contact with the cornea when the device has already been in contact with the cornea of another person, unless required, because of a theoretical risk of transmitting the variant Creutzfeldt–Jakob disease (vCJD) prion. This was based on advice given by SEAC, the Spongiform Encephalopathy Advisory Committee, to Department of Health (DoH) in 1999.

The College of Optometrists and Association of British Dispensing Opticians have recommended guidelines for sterilization in response to the warning. However, the recommended decontamination procedure (1 hour in 2% sodium hypochlorite solution followed with rinsing in sterile saline) is only for RGP contact lenses. The efficacy of the procedure for sterilization of other instruments is still under research. Therefore, while this advice is still in place and alternative noncontact methods are available, these lenses are generally confined to the back of the drawer.

Indirect ophthalmoscopy

Slit-lamp binocular indirect ophthalmoscopy (BIO)

This technique has gained huge popularity in recent times, such that many practitioners have incorporated the use of hand-held indirect lenses to view the fundus into their general routine. Indirect lenses are high-plus lenses that are used in conjunction with a slit-lamp to produce a virtual image of the fundus that is laterally reversed and inverted. Therefore the clinician that is new to this technique has to adjust their observation to account for an upside-down, mirror image.

There are a number of lenses available on the market. They are available with a number of modifications. These include:

- yellow filters – that are either fixed or detachable. This reduces the amount of blue light impacting on the fundus, which is important in prolonged examinations
- lid adapters – that help separate the lids and set the lens at the correct working distance
- graticules – that are useful for measuring
- mounts – which steady the lens on the slit lamp.

The best field of view is obtained by the higher dioptric powered lenses, but at a compromise to working distance. Each lens produces a stereoscopic fundus view that is only marginally magnified, with the greatest magnification being achieved with the lower powers. The slit-lamp's observation system is utilized to increase the magnification of the image. Table 7.2 lists some of the properties of lenses that are commercially available. The information has been collated from the manufacturers data.

Examination technique

- For the best results, the pupil is dilated with an appropriate pharmaceutical agent(s).
- The patient is instructed on the need for maximum compliance and asked to fixate the slit-lamp fixation target.
- The microscope is placed in the straight-ahead position with the lamp coaxial (allowing binocular viewing). The magnification is set to its lowest position and slit adjusted to a height around 5 mm and width 3–4 mm.
- The slit is focused on the patient's cornea and centered. The lens is introduced close to the patient's eye (Figure 7.3). The lens can be held either way around.
- The slit lamp is focused by moving it toward the patient, past the inverted image of the patient's pupil/iris until an image of the retina is seen (Figure 7.4).

Table 7.2 A comparison of the different hand-held indirect lenses

Power (D)	Magnification	Field of view (°)	Working distance form the cornea (mm)	Indications for use
60	1.15×	76	11	Disc and macula
78	0.93×	84	8	General screening
90	0.75×	94	6	General screening. Works well with small pupils
SuperField	0.76×	95	7	General screening. Works well with small pupils
Variable zoom	0.77–0.94×	78–100	5	General screening
132 SP	0.45×	99	4	Wide field, small pupils

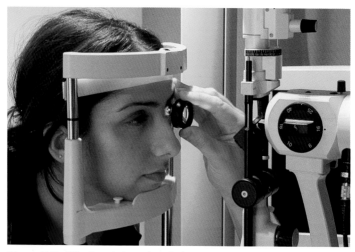

Figure 7.3 The lens is introduced close to the patient's eye

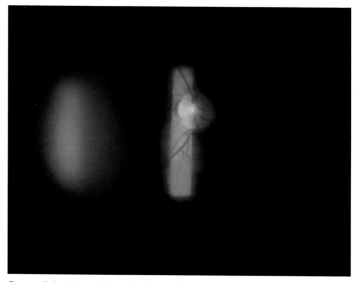

Figure 7.4 The slit lamp is focused by moving it toward the patient, past the inverted image of the patient's pupil/iris until an image of the retina is seen

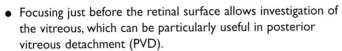

- Focusing just before the retinal surface allows investigation of the vitreous, which can be particularly useful in posterior vitreous detachment (PVD).
- By bringing the lens closer to the eye the field of view can be increased. Any reflections from the slit lamp can be minimized or eliminated by slightly tilting the lens either vertically or horizontally.
- The image can be optimized by adjusting the magnification and slit width/height on the slit lamp.
- The eye is examined in various positions of gaze. The lens is repositioned each time to optimize the view. If the observer requires the image to move then the lens is moved in the same direction as the desired movement.

Slit-lamp BIO can be used to examine a patient with undilated pupils. The lenses, which are specifically designed for use on a small pupil, work best in these instances. Nonetheless, a good view of the disk can be obtained in most patients. BIO has many advantages but also has some significant disadvantages, these are listed in Table 7.3.

Table 7.3 **Benefits and pitfalls of slit-lamp BIO**

Advantages	Disadvantages
Wide field of view making it easy to scan fundus	Image is virtual, laterally reversed and inverted
Image degrades significantly less with media opacities compared with direct methods	Magnification and image quality limited by slit-lamp
Excellent in detecting stereoscopic and color changes	Difficult to use on small pupils
Inexpensive (assuming slit-lamp is available)	Difficult to use on noncompliant patients
Magnification does not vary with patient's refractive error	Unsuitable for domiciliary work, patient has to be upright

(continued)

Table 7.3 **Continued**

Advantages	Disadvantages
Comfortable distance from patient maintained	Needs a lot of practice to become proficient
	Can be uncomfortable for the patient
	Reflections reduce image quality
	Scanning required to build full picture

Headborne binocular indirect ophthalmoscopy

The headset BIO is used in conjunction with a condensing lens and best results are obtained when the pupil is maximally dilated. The condensing lens collects the image of the retina from the patient's eye. The optometrist views this image binocularly (Figure 7.5). Greatest magnification is achieved with a low-powered condensing lens; however, this compromises the field of view. Higher-powered lenses have to be held closer to the patient.

The field of view that is produced is approximately 10× wider than that achieved with direct ophthalmoscopy. The binoculaur viewing conditions ensure good stereopsis and there is negligible change in magnification with the patient's refractive error. The image produced by a headset BIO is laterally reversed and

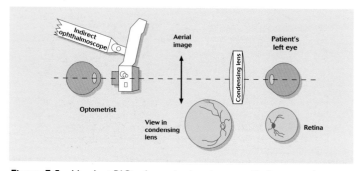

Figure 7.5 Headset BIO schematic showing magnified, reversed, inverted image. Courtesy of David Austen

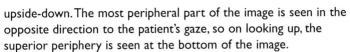
upside-down. The most peripheral part of the image is seen in the opposite direction to the patient's gaze, so on looking up, the superior periphery is seen at the bottom of the image.

The wide field of view produced by this technique makes it ideal for examining the peripheral fundus, however, its low magnification can lead to subtle changes or small lesions being missed.

Modified (monocular) indirect ophthalmoscopy

Examination of an uncooperative patient is difficult. Many of the techniques described above require patient compliance. The direct ophthalmoscope generally offers the best solution, but it too has a difficulty – patients often fret as the clinician approaches and moreover, the patient is most likely to fixate the ophthalmoscope light. This generally results in good view of the fovea and macula but little else!

The direct ophthalmoscope can be used in conjunction with a condensing lens (the condensing lens in the headset BIO is ideal, see Figure 7.6). This provides the observer with a moderately

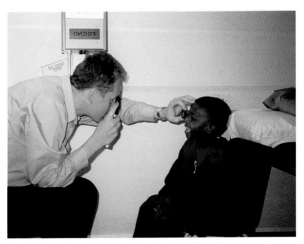

Figure 7.6 Modified (monocular) indirect ophthalmoscopy (reproduced with permission from Doshi & Harvey *Investigative Techniques and Ocular Examination*, Butterworth-Heinemann 2003)

magnified and wider-angle view of the posterior pole. An inverted, laterally reversed image is produced. A magnification of 4–5× is achieved which can be increased slightly by the practitioner moving closer. It also allows the clinician to work at 20–50 cm from the patient, thus allowing for the anxious patient.

This technique is particularly useful for viewing the central fundus in children and with practice the practitioner is able to get a reasonable view of the disk and macula. The main disadvantage of this technique is the lack of stereopsis. However, lateral movement to induce parallax, can provide clues to depth perception.

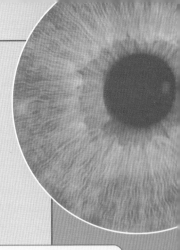

8
Ocular
photography

Introduction

All clinicians are taught to document any interesting features that they may encounter during the course of their examination of a patient. In its most rudimentary form this often is a sketch of the area of concern. Although seemingly useful this process is not without flaw. Errors occur in the representation of a lesion and it is often difficult for a practitioner to meaningfully determine what a colleague is trying to represent.

The use of photography has long been advocated as a superior alternative to a basic diagram. However, in the past the delay between taking the photographs, processing the film and viewing the final results have generally made it impractical. Additionally, the significant expense (which is increased if the whole process needed to be repeated) has meant that this has rarely taken-off within the mainstream of the optical profession, with most of the photography being confined to hospital eye departments.

Digital imaging and powerful computers have become part of our everyday lives and as such it is perhaps not surprising that these advances have been widely adopted by the ophthalmic profession. The introduction of this technology to image and record the whole of the eye has revolutionized ocular photography and with ever-reducing prices, ocular-imaging systems are now becoming relatively commonplace in general optical practice. For example, to participate in diabetic screening, the National Screening Committee requires digital fundus camera imaging.

The purpose of this chapter is to introduce the reader to the concepts of digital imaging. For the enthusiast, an excellent book by James Wolfsohn in the *Eye Essentials* series concentrates on this very subject.

Hardware considerations

Digital cameras have one of three types of light-detection systems (or chips). The first two are the most commonly used in ophthalmic imaging devices. The chips are:

- CCD (charged couple device). This is the most well known and consists of etched pixels on a metal oxide semiconductor made from silicone. The pixels convert light that falls upon them into electrons. They sense the amount of light rather than its color. Photon to electron conversion occurs on the pixel, allowing a maximum amount of space to remain on the pixel for light-capturing information. They therefore have a low signal-to-noise ratio. The electron to voltage conversion is done on the chip leaving the supporting camera circuit to digitize this analog data.

- CMOS (complementary metal oxide semi-conductor). These are similar to CCDs but both the photon-electron and electron-voltage is conducted within the pixel together with digitization of the signal. As a result there is less room on the light-sensitive part of the sensor, consequently a microlens is used to capture more light within the pixel area and bend it towards the light-sensitive part of the pixel. These chips are usually cheaper than CCDs.

- Foveon. This is a chip of transparent quartz that contains three layers of CMOS embedded in silicon, positioned to take advantage of the fact that silicon absorbs light of different wavelengths at different depths. This should enable each pixel to be able to record individual values for green, red and blue. These chips are less common and are currently held back by technical problems

Fixed CCD or CMOS chips contain a grid of light-sensitive pixels that can only capture light levels rather than color information. Therefore to capture a colored image cameras used in slit-lamp photography use one of two techniques. The first is to coat each pixel in a different primary color (red, green or blue), spatially arranged in a mosaic pattern. The image processing takes the intensity level into account when determining the color of an individual pixel, resulting in an image at the full resolution of the chip but with only 90–95% spectral fidelity. This can result in color fringing around the sharp edges.

The second technique is to utilize three chips rather than one, with each capturing an image at its full resolution but

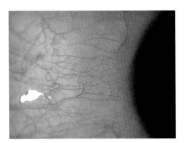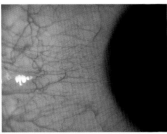

Figure 8.1 Image produced by a single chip camera (left) and three chip camera (right) (Images courtesy of James Wolfsohn)

through a different filter (red, green or blue). Prisms behind the lens allow green filtered light to pass undiverted to their chip, whereas red and blue light is diverted to their respective chip. The processing converts the image to resolution of one chip allowing for absolute data for red, green and blue and therefore allowing for 100% spatial and spectral fidelity (compare the images for a single chip and three-chip camera in Figure 8.1). These cameras require more light than single chip cameras for an equivalent image.

Optical and light considerations

In order to achieve an excellent photograph it is essential that the optics of the system producing the image (for the camera to capture) are of the highest caliber. As a result of the small capture size area of the chip (compared with 35 mm film) image quality is of the essence. As well as stating the type of chip used the size of the chip should also be recorded. A pixel receptor will be larger on a larger chip of the same resolution as a smaller chip. The larger the pixel receptor target the more chance a photon has of hitting it. Digital cameras boasting resolutions around 6 megapixels on a 12 mm chip have pixel

receptors <1 μm in diameter and are therefore limited by the
size of a photon.

Additional lighting is essential for optometric digital imaging
due to light being lost from intervening beamsplitters, lenses,
incomplete fill factor of the sensor pixels and reduced light
sensitivity compared to the human eye. This is particularly the
case for cobalt blue photography as CCDs and CMOSs are most
responsive at the red end of the spectrum. These chips therefore
often have infrared filters and compensate for low blue sensitivity
blue signals during the image processing. Many of the currently
available commercial systems have external illuminators to
provide the extra light needed during photography.

Image transfer and storage

Once an image has been taken it needs to be transferred
from the camera to the computer for storage. Transfer can
occur manually by moving the memory card from camera to
computer but more commonly occurs via an analog, USB or
firewire cable. Using the latter method speeds up the process
of image transfer.

Reducing the number of colors has a significant effect on the
file size. An 8-bit color can code 256 colors for each pixel. High
color (12-bit) can code 65536 colors and true color (24-bit)
16777216. An uncompressed 800 by 600 pixel 24-bit takes up
1.44 Mb of storage space. Therefore, when taking images it is
important to consider their use. Low resolution may be
acceptable for patient education, but high resolution will be
required when monitoring or screening pathology (see Figure 8.2).

Most systems offer different formats to save images and
movies. These are summarized in Table 8.1.

Anterior segment photographic systems

Photography of the anterior segment can be achieved by one
of two methods – either via an eyepiece attachment or an

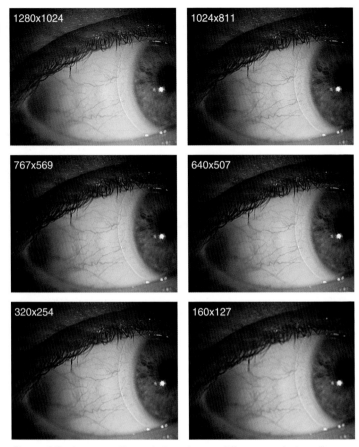

Figure 8.2 Image quality varieties taken at different resolutions (Images courtesy of James Wolfsohn)

internal beamsplitter. Eyepiece attachments have the main advantage in that they are relatively cheap, however, it is important to remember that there is always going to be additional costs for software and the extra hardware that will be required.

Table 8.1 **File formats**

Abbreviated name	Full name	Functions/usage
TIF	Tagged information file	Stores all data (no loss) once internal processing has taken place. It uses algorithms to make file smaller for storage but these are reversed on opening the file. Images that are stored are relatively large – a 1600 × 1200 pixel image in 24-bit color approximates to a 5.8 Mb TIF
JPEG	Joint photographic experts group	A compressed format resulting in the loss of some image quality. JPEG compression attempts to eliminate redundant or non-necessary information. RGB files are converted to luminance and chrominance components, merging pixels and utilizing compression algorithms on 8 × 8 pixel blocks removing frequencies not used by the human eye. Different compression levels can be selected (see Figure 8.3). For example a 1600 × 1200 pixel in 24-bit color with low-compression JPEG approximates to 0.3 Mb
RAW		A new format allowing data to be stored in its raw form before any processing takes place. This results in smaller files than in TIF format and the archived data are available for reprocessing. This requires proprietary software to convert the image to a readable format
BMP	Bitmap	Most commonly used as an uncompressed format and as such the resultant files are rather large

(continued)

Table 8.1 **Continued**

Abbreviated name	Full name	Functions/usage
AVI (movie files)	Audio video interleave	Audio and video files are interleaved such that the information can be stored consecutively or as separate streams
MPEG (movie files)	Moving pictures experts group	MPEG defines a compressed bit data stream. The compression algorithm varies with individual manufacturers. MPEG uses many of the same techniques as JPEG but adds interframe compression to exploit similarities that occur between successive frames

For an eyepiece-based system the normal configuration of the slit-lamp eyepieces has to be reversed. Therefore, the optical path is different to that of a dedicated photographic slit-lamp. Light loss occurs at the eyepiece lens assembly but an internal beamsplitter is unnecessary. In these types of system the field of view is generally reduced and moreover the camera normally obscures at least one of the eyepieces, thus making alignment and focusing more difficult.

The second option for anterior segment photography is to place a beamsplitter into the optical path of the slit-lamp. Most photo-slit-lamps currently on the market are of this form. A beamsplitter module can be added to most medium- to high-quality slit-lamps. The beamsplitter can be dropped into place when photography is required but removed when a general examination is necessary. The use of a beamsplitter still allows binocular viewing through the eyepieces but the camera receives only about 50% of the available light.

For a comparison of the different anterior segment imaging systems available the reader is referred to the dedicated book by James Wolfsohn on this subject.

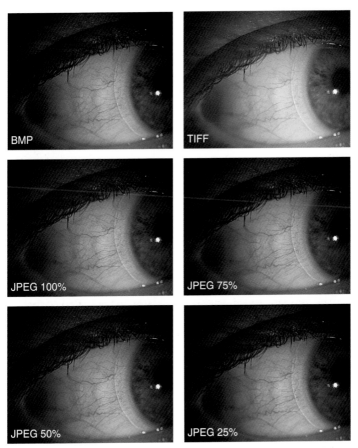

Figure 8.3 The effect of compression on image quality (Image courtesy of James Wolfsohn)

Retinal photographic systems

Traditional film-based camera systems have now been superseded by digital imaging systems as a result of the former's high costs and long waiting times between image acquisition and being able to view the final image. Both factors were increased if a poor image was obtained and the process had to be repeated.

Most modern retinal cameras use digital imaging, allowing images to be viewed instantaneously. This offers the benefit of immediate determination of the most appropriate luminance to be used and enables the viewer to optimize the image before capture. It is interesting to note that currently the National Screening Committee recommends the use of digital photography for diabetic screening, although there are conflicting opinions in this debate.

Retinal cameras image the fundus initially as a black-and-white image to allow for alignment. A high-powered positive lens is then dropped into place to neutralize the power of the lens and the cornea, allowing an inverted aerial image of the fundus to be seen. This is also normally a black-and-white image as the lack of filters to allow color image processing enables an image with lower light levels.

As with anterior segment systems, the optics of the camera is essential to gain a high-quality image. However, the fundus image is also reliant on the optics of the eye, any media opacities or corneal irregularities. In such cases dilatation will be of benefit. The image obtained will be dependent on the patient's refractive error and this can vary with each camera. This has been found to vary between 5 to 30%. This can affect measurements taken. Moreover, the ability to monitor a lesion may be affected if different cameras are used over a duration of time.

Once alignment has been achieved with the black-and-white image, capture is achieved with a color camera and the fundus is illuminated for this purpose with a flash. Complete color control of the image is essential to highlight important features such as blood vessels, hemorrhages and pigment lesions. Often the camera takes the raw information regarding the amount of light falling on each pixel location and processes this before storing it in an image file (usually in TIF format).

The National Screening Committee has determined that the minimum pixel resolution for diabetic screening is currently 20 pixels per degree and that no image compression should occur. However, research has suggested that a compressed JPEG

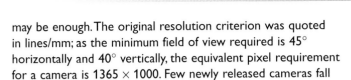
may be enough. The original resolution criterion was quoted in lines/mm; as the minimum field of view required is 45° horizontally and 40° vertically, the equivalent pixel requirement for a camera is 1365 × 1000. Few newly released cameras fall below these resolution and field requirements.

For a comparison of the different retinal segment imaging systems available the reader is referred to the dedicated book on this subject.

This chapter is based on the series of articles published in *Optician* listed below.

Further reading

Wolfsohn J, Petersen H Technology, Part 1: Optometric imaging systems. *Optician* **227**: 26–29.

Wolfsohn J, Petersen H Slit lamp systems, Part 2: Optometric imaging systems. *Optician* **227**: 16–21.

Wolfsohn J, Petersen H (2004) Slit lamp photography: Instrument Insight. *Optometry Today*

Wolfsohn J, Petersen H, Bartlett H Retinal Imaging systems, Part 3: Optometric imaging systems. *Optician* **227**: 18–24.

9
Essentials of visual field assessment

Introduction

The investigation of the visual field is an essential component of any eye examination as it may detect both early ocular and neurological disease processes which other investigations may miss. Detailed and accurate field screening or investigation is a subject covered in depth in a sister book in this series (see *Visual Fields* by Robert Cubbidge).

The extent of the absolute visual field is dependent upon the shape of the head of the patient, but it is important to remember that the extent of the temporal field is almost always greater than 90°. Typical values are 100° temporally, 75° inferiorly, and 60° nasally and superiorly. The last two are most patient dependent because of variable nose and brow size.

Binocularly, the two monocular visual fields overlap, resulting in a stereoscopic zone which is approximately 120° in the horizontal dimension. The extreme temporal periphery of the binocular field is seen monocularly. The retinal image of the visual field is upside down and back to front. Therefore, the projection of the visual field is such that the superior visual field corresponds to the inferior retina and vice versa. Similarly, the temporal component of the visual field corresponds to the nasal retina and vice versa.

Static or kinetic

It is well understood that the retinal sensitivity to any target decreases the further away from the fovea the image falls. This was classically described by Traquair as representing a hill of vision whose peak corresponded to the fovea and whose slopes represented the gradual reduction in sensitivity towards the periphery of the retina until 'the sea of blindness' is reached; the point beyond which no target presented will be seen.

Kinetic perimetry involves the movement of a constant sized target from beyond the field of vision to the point where it is just seen. The larger target should be seen closer to the extent of the absolute field, the smaller target further to the center of the field. In this way, kinetic perimetry may define the 'hill of vision' by the use of variously sized targets moved to the point of identification. Generally, kinetic perimetry is primarily used in gross assessment of the visual field when a quick test is needed to detect a major scotoma or cause of constricted field.

Static perimetry employs the use of a target or targets (multiple stimulus or tachistoscopic presentation) of increasing intensity presented to the same point or points within a field until the intensity is reached at which the target is just seen. The majority of automated central visual field screeners employ multiple static stimulus presentation as it is more repeatable, often quicker, and more useful for defining more subtle scotoma as well as allowing for the depth of a partial or relative scotoma (that is, a blind spot where vision is maintained but at a reduced level). Less controlled gross variations of static perimetry are also useful, such as some of the confrontation tests used in neurology or the Amsler grid.

Confrontation

Though the terms confrontation and gross perimetry are often used as synonyms, strictly speaking confrontation describes one of several 'comparison' tests whereas gross perimetry is the use of a target to measure the extent of the visual field and to map any large scotomas within the field. One form of confrontation involves the use of a target moved along an imaginary flat plane between and perpendicular to the gaze of the patient and the practitioner. This obviously will not allow the temporal extent of field to be measured, but will allow the practitioner to confirm that any areas they see can also be seen by the patient. One could also describe other tests as confrontation tests, for example, the presentation of two red targets to the hemifields of the patient to find out whether one of the targets is desaturated, or the use of a shiny coin in four quadrants of the field of one eye. Many confrontation tests are used by neurologists in investigating possible neurological lesions.

Gross perimetry

Gross perimetry describes the use of a handheld target held at a constant distance from the patient's eye which, when brought in an arc from beyond their visual field boundary, allows them to announce when the target is first seen (the extent of field or boundary for that particular target size and color). When the target is moved further within their field to the central point of fixation allows any large defect to be detected.

The choice of target dictates the extent of the isopter, just as with any kinetic assessment. A larger target will be seen at a greater eccentricity, while the isopter for a small target will be contracted. Similarly, a white target brought from beyond the field will be seen before a red target which will itself be seen before a green target. In practice, though a small white target might be justifiable in terms of sensitivity, a red target is generally chosen as it will contrast better with typical wall coverings within the consulting room. To maintain some degree of correlation with a 5 mm white target (typical for gross perimetry), a 15 mm diameter red target may be used instead, its extra size counteracting the reduced sensitivity to red compared to white.

The Amsler chart

The Amsler chart represents a simple method of assessing the quality of the central field of vision. The test includes several charts, the basic and most commonly used being a square white grid printed on a dull black background comprising 20 rows and 20 columns of smaller squares (Figure 9.1).

When viewed at 28 cm, each square subtends 1° at the retina. The grid therefore is used to assess the field 10° either side of the fixation point when viewed monocularly (as should always be the case). It is, therefore, only possible to map out the physiological blind spot by directing the patient to view the nasal edge of the grid such that the blind spot 15° temporal to this point falls onto the grid. Though rarely done, it is in theory

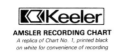

AMSLER RECORDING CHART
*A replica of Chart No. 1, printed black
on white for convenience of recording*

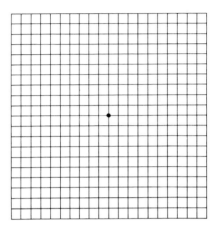

KEELER LIMITED
Clewer Hill Road, Windsor Berkshire SL4 4AA
Tel: (01753) 857177 Telex: 847565 Fax: (01753) 857817

Figure 9.1 The Amsler recording grid chart is useful for detecting central defects in the macular area

possible to detect blind spot extension in, for example, myelinated nerve fibers around the disk or in early papilloedema. Typically, however, the grid is used to assess macular function.

Indications for its use include the following:

- evidence of macular disturbance seen on ophthalmoscopy in either eye (if seen in just one eye, both eyes require investigation because of the bilateral nature of most macular diseases)
- unexplainable loss of central visual acuity

- reduction of acuity through a pinhole
- symptoms of central visual disturbance, such as distortion
- history of systemic disease or more commonly drugs which may predispose to a maculopathy (such as tamoxifen or chloroquine). For the assessment of possible early toxic maculopathy, the red Amsler grid may be slightly more sensitive
- for the mapping of a central scotoma already detected. This is useful for monitoring any progression of a scotoma. For this assessment, the grid with diagonal cross lines is useful to encourage stable fixation. The patient should be asked to fixate upon the point where they imagine the center of the cross to be. In cases of poor performance with magnification, noting the position of the scotoma relative to the center is useful. A scotoma shifted towards the right of the field will have a greater impact upon the ability to scan from left to right when reading
- history of poor photo stress recovery. Reports of persistent after images after exposure to, for example, a flashlight or difficulty in adapting to changes in ambient light levels may indicate early macular disease.

A simple procedure might be as follows:

- Correct the patient to adequately see the target at 28 cm. Illumination should be good without constituting a glare source, and one eye should be occluded.
- The patient should be directed to fixate upon the dot in the center of the grid. As poor fixation is perhaps the main source of error in any field assessment, this instruction cannot be repeated enough throughout the test.
- While looking at the central target, the patient should report if any of the four corners of the grid are missing and, if so, the missing area should be shaded on the record sheet (a replica grid only in black on a white background).
- The patient should then report if any of the grid is missing and, if so, the position and size of the blind spot noted.

- The patient should then report if any of the lines are wavy or distorted and again this should be recorded if found. If distorted, it is useful to note if the distortion is static (as might be the case with an old atrophic scar or a heavy concentration of drusen around the fovea) or moving or shimmering. The latter, described as metamorphopsia, might be indicative of an active exudative process (such as prior to choroidal neovascularization) and might warrant an urgent referral.

In cases where one eye has already suffered macular disease, or where there is evidence of macular disturbance yet to affect vision, many practitioners give a copy of the grid to the patient who may then self-monitor their central field on a regular basis at home and in the knowledge that they must report any new disturbance they might detect.

Sensitivity versus specificity

So far, the assessments considered have been fairly crude. Their ability to detect minor changes in the field of vision are limited (so have a low sensitivity). On the other hand, any defect detected is likely to be actual and related to an abnormal process (so their specificity is high). The balance of the ability to detect disease while on the other hand ensuring that no patients without disease fail the test (so the balance between sensitivity and specificity) is an important one for field assessment and the relationship between the two may be changed according to the desired outcome. An incredibly bright target should be seen by all normally sighted people and only those with a significant defect would miss it. This would represent maximum specificity which is usually defined as a percentage (in this case 100%). On the other hand, most people with even a mild field defect would still report seeing the light and so many early-disease presentations would be missed (low sensitivity).

The highest sensitivity would be gained by using stimuli of an intensity just visible to the point of the retina to which it is presented and which would not be seen if of a lower intensity.

This form of presentation is described as a full-threshold assessment as it employs stimuli of an intensity set at the threshold of the retinal ability to detect them. This maximum sensitivity should allow even the mildest partial scotoma to be detected. However, many normals might also struggle to see some of the stimuli and report them as missing. This therefore would represent low specificity. Generally speaking, a screening program should be sensitive to detect most eye disease while specific enough for normals to pass the assessment. A suprathreshold assessment uses stimuli of a set intensity brighter than the threshold such that all normals should see them and yet defects of a depth greater than the intensity level above threshold should fail the assessment.

Generally for screening purposes, a suprathreshold assessment is preferred as it is quicker, sensitive enough to detect most defects while allowing most normals to pass. For investigation of a suspicious patient presentation, such as someone with glaucomatous disk appearance or a strong family history of glaucoma, a full-threshold assessment, though more demanding of the patient, is more likely to detect even the first evidence of reduced retinal function.

Automated field screeners

Most automated field screeners assess the central field to within 25–30° from fixation. Though it is true that around 85% of field defects fall within this space, the remaining minority affecting the intermediate and far periphery are often greatly clinically significant. Such defects might result from retinal damage, as with, for example, chorioretinitis, retinal detachment, a neoplasm or early retinitis pigmentosa. It is also important to remember that many defects due to damage to the visual pathway may also start in the far periphery and only extend into the central field at a later stage. An example might be the superior bitemporal loss due to compression of the chiasma from below by a pituitary adenoma. A gross perimetry assessment is always worthwhile, therefore, to support a more accurate automated static central assessment. Some of the screeners do, however, allow the practitioner to select a program which does assess further away from the center, such as the Dicon or the Zeiss Humphrey Visual Field Analyzer.

Most modern screeners establish the threshold sensitivity at each point to which a stimulus is presented, though many machines in general practice (such as older Henson models) are usually used at a suprathreshold setting for speed. The Humphrey Visual Field Analyzer may be programed to assess the field faster by incorporating the Swedish Interactive Thresholding Algorithm. It was designed as an attempt to decrease the time taken for a traditional staircase method assessment (a 4–2dB algorithm typically takes 15 minutes) yet maintaining good sensitivity in glaucoma detection. Time is reduced in several ways as the algorithm specifies the appropriate stimulus brightness to be presented at each point, may monitor the time of response to adopt appropriate subsequent presentations, and is able to stop once sufficient information has been taken. The presentation of stimuli at levels around that at which 50% are seen greatly reduces the speed of testing. So by better pacing of the test, and the useful interpretation of false positives and false negatives, the SITA appears to correlate well with standard perimetric assessment yet in less time. The reduced timing is likely to help accuracy of patient response. Longer does not necessarily mean better with field assessment as poor compliance, fatigue and loss of fixation all play an increasing part in reducing the accuracy of field assessment. This is one of the reasons why it is essential, if a field defect is suspected, for the test to be repeated to ensure that it is not artefactual.

Reliability indices

As already stated, one of the major problems with field assessment is the detection of abnormal data that is due to patient 'error', such as poor fixation or fatigue leading to points reported as seen when actually missed (a false positive) and vice versa (false negative). Many modern screeners, such as the

Humphrey VFA or the Oculus easy field, record these errors such that the reliability of a plot might be interpreted by a practitioner. A common method of assessing fixation loss is by using the Heijl–Krakau technique method of monitoring fixation throughout a field assessment by means of projecting a stimulus to an assumed location of the blind spot. If fixation is not present, the patient will respond to this stimulus and the machine will note the number of errors. The technique relies upon an estimate as to the exact anatomical location of the optic disc, so is open to error. Other instruments use gaze tracking which allows a continual assessment of fixation throughout by monitoring the relative positions of every stimulus presented. False positives are recorded when a stimulus which has not been shown or has been presented at an intensity known to be below the threshold value for the individual is still reported as seen. A false negative is recorded when a stimulus known to have been previously seen is now missed. Any significant score in the reliability indices is an indication that the assessment needs to be repeated, usually on another occasion, as the plot cannot be usefully interpreted and acted upon.

Total and pattern deviation

Some instruments, notably the Humphrey VFA, incorporate software allowing analysis of any variation in the assessed field. Any threshold value found to be below that expected in an age-matched population will show up as a defect in the total deviation plot. Fogging a 20-year-old normal patient will reduce their threshold value across the entire field and this would show up as an extensive total deviation. A similar effect is seen with, for example, cataract.

The pattern deviation plot represents significant variation in retinal sensitivity within the field, as might be the case with a scotoma. If a patient has a cataract and also glaucoma, it is possible that they have an extensive total deviation defect while just the earliest signs of an arcuate defect in the pattern deviation plot. In this way, the screener actually has some diagnostic value.

Interpreting field defects

Every field screener produces its own particular plot and interpretation varies depending upon the model. This is covered in much greater detail in *Visual Fields Eye Essentials* by Robert Cubbidge. However, a few general points should be outlined.

- Any repeatable defect needs to be taken seriously. If not repeatable or if the reliability indices, where available, suggest poor patient response, then other investigations may be needed before a management plan initiated.
- Overall threshold values between the eyes should be similar. If not, this may indicate reduced light levels reaching the retina, as with media opacification.
- Single points of reduced sensitivity close to the disc often represent the obscuration of photoreceptors by an overlying retinal blood vessel (an angioscotoma).
- Defects found in the area between the blind spot and fixation (centrocecal defects) usually are associated with damage to the papillomacular bundle of retinal nerve fibers as can occur with toxic responses to drugs or excessive alcohol consumption.
- Field loss in one eye is due to a lesion anterior to the optic chiasma.
- Irregular, asymmetric loss in both eyes which does not seem to be limited by the horizontal or vertical midlines is often related to focal retinal damage and can be confirmed by ophthalmoscopy.
- Progressive optic neuropathy, such as glaucoma, will tend to affect the arcuate fibers initially (usually inferior first as there is a greater susceptibility to damage here) resulting in an arcuate defect. The arcuate fibers extend temporally to the fovea to end at the horizontal raphe (Figure 9.2).

This represents the boundary between the superior and inferior nerve tissues from embryological development. Superior and inferior arcuate loss often ends at different positions at this temporal boundary, and the resultant step in the nasal field is significant evidence of arcuate fiber damage.

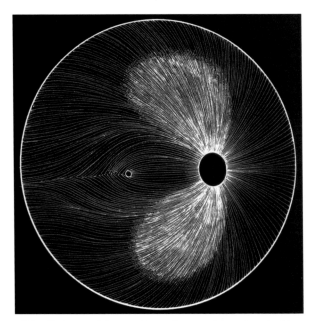

Figure 9.2 Pathway of the ganglion cell axons (reproduced with permission from Litwak *Glaucoma Handbook*, Butterworth-Heinemann 2001)

- Any defect clearly respecting the horizontal midline is likely to be retinal in cause. If sudden onset, this is most likely a vascular incident, as with the altitudinal defect in Figure 9.3.
- Any defect respecting the vertical midline is likely to be due to damage within the visual pathway from the chiasma or behind.
- Heteronymous loss is due to chiasmal damage, either due to pressure on the nasal fibers as with the bitemporal loss due to pituitary adenoma, or on the temporal fibers, as with the binasal loss due to an internal carotid aneurysm.
- Damage to the visual pathway posterior to the chiasma results in homonymous loss. This will be more symmetrical (or congruous) the further back in the pathway the lesion is, increasing significantly in congruence posterior to the lateral geniculate nuclei.

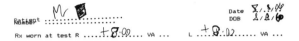

HENSON CFA3000   Tinsley

Patient
Number ....

Rx worn at test R ....+8.00... VA ...   L ...+8.02...... VA ...

Date ...
DOB ...

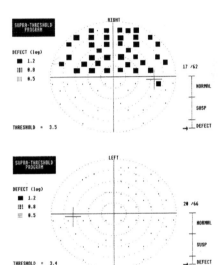

Figure 9.3 Altitudinal defects are typical in retinal or vascular based pathology

- The optic radiations spread through two major lobes of the brain, the parietal and temporal. A common site for damage due to a cerebrovascular accident, damage to the radiations in a patient who survives stroke often leaves a homonymous quadranopic defect.
- Damage to the occipital lobe may result in a homonymous hemianopia.

As a significant number of nerve fibers are damaged before detectable field loss results, any repeatable field defect must be treated as important and would usually warrant referral. In the case of a lesion in the visual pathway, this may be an urgent or emergency referral (as with the binasal defect mentioned above).

Adapted assessment for early-stage glaucoma

Much research has suggested that there is selective nerve fiber damage in glaucoma, with the magnocellular pathway being affected before the parvocellular pathway. Attempts have been made to use stimuli to which the receptors attached to magnocellular ganglion cell fibers are particularly receptive, in an attempt to detect field loss in glaucoma at an earlier stage. Short-wave automated perimetry (SWAP) is one such attempt (as may be introduced to a Humphrey VFA or the Octopus) which uses short-wavelength stimuli thought to be magnocellular responsive.

Another method employs the presentation to various parts of the field a sine grating that alternates in shade repeatedly such that the spatial frequency is seen to double. The ability to detect this so-called frequency doubling is again thought to reduce in early glaucoma and so the Zeiss Humphrey FDT may be used in specific glaucoma screening programs.

Further reading

Flanagan JG (1998) Glaucoma update: epidemiology and new approaches to medical management. *Ophthalmic Physiol Opt* **18**: 126–138.

Lawrenson J (1997) Anatomy and physiology of aqueous production and drainage. In: *Continuing Professional Development–Glaucoma*, Ch 1. Association of Optometrists/Optometry Today: Fleet.

McAllister JA and Wilson RP (1986) *Glaucoma*. Butterworths: Oxford.

O'Kelly H and Macnaughton J (1997) Examination of the glaucomatous eye. In: *Continuing Professional Development–Glaucoma*, Ch 5 Association of Optometrists/Optometry Today: Fleet.

Pointer JS (1997) The diurnal variation of intraocular pressure in non-glaucomatous subjects: relevance in a clinical context. *Ophthalmic Physiol Opt* **17**: 456–465.

Ruskell G (1997) Intraocular pressure variations in glaucoma. In: *Continuing Professional Development–Glaucoma*, Ch 9. Association of Optometrists/Optometry Today: Fleet.

Tielsch JM (1991) A population-based evaluation of glaucoma screening: the Baltimore Eye Survey. *Am J Epidemiol* **134**: 1102–1110.

10
Advanced instrumentation

Introduction

Advances in technology have led to improvements in methods of measuring and assessing ocular structures. The increasing use of the laser has developed alongside microprocessor improvements allowing miniaturization of hardware and improved software capability. Increasingly, much of the optometric assessment may be automated and digital encoding of clinical data allows accurate storage, measurement and analysis. While this chapter is necessarily a brief overview of such technology (both because of the limited space in a book such as this as well as the rapid advances making in-depth discussion rapidly outdated), it is important to recognize the increasing role of technology in optometry.

Scanning laser ophthalmoscopy

The confocal scanning technique was introduced around 1980 by Petran and Boyde and has been adopted in many clinical and biological fields. The basic principle involves the production of a collimated polarized laser beam which is deflected stepwise across the two x and y-directions by a scanning unit. The continually deflecting beam is then reflected by a dichroic mirror (the beamsplitter) to pass through the objective lens which focuses the light to the point at the level to be viewed. Light emitted from the target reaches the beam-splitter again which remains transparent to the selected wavelength from the target point, while eliminating all out-of-focus light (from points above or below the target point). The x-y deflection allows this to be done for all points in a plane at the established level and, by doing this for a variety of planes, a sequence of 'slices' through the object viewed may be imaged. The wavelength of the beam will be important in terms of its penetration of whatever is being viewed.

The main advantage of this system is that it can be used to carry out retinal investigations in ways that enable the

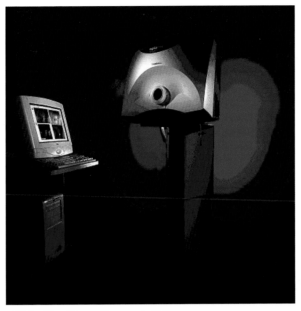

Figure 10.1 The Optos Panoramic 200

ophthalmologist or optometrist to gain more information about the retina than can be obtained from conventional imaging techniques.

The Optos Panoramic 200 (Figure 10.1) is designed to enable an area of up to 200° of the fundus to be produced as one image and without the use of collaging or pupil dilation. The SLO tends to be superior to standard imaging methods when cataract is present and can be used for both fluorescein and indocyanine green angiography.

The large field image produced by the Panoramic combined with the unfamiliar coloring often takes some experience to interpret. Indeed the instrument initially led to an increase in referrals of eyes subsequently found to be within healthy bounds. However, the improved view of the peripheral fundus (Figure 10.2), remarkably in an undilated eye, has improved the clinician's ability to detect and manage peripheral retinal disease.

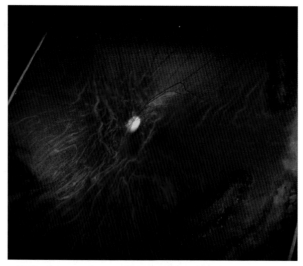

Figure 10.2 Improved view of the peripheral fundus by the Panoramic 200 allows greater accuracy in detecting peripheral lesions

Scanning laser polarimetry

By its simplest definition, a polarimeter is an instrument capable of measuring either the polarity (unidirectional property of light) or rotations to that polarity. As light passes through a structure, the nature of the change to the light gives information about the properties of that structure.

Layered structures may exhibit properties not found when the individual materials are assessed. An example of this is when waves traversing a medium, with their electric fields perpendicular to the medium, experience a different index of refraction than the waves parallel to the plane of the medium. This difference is due to the varying boundary conditions imposed on the electric fields parallel and perpendicular to the interfaces between the different layers. This property is known as birefringence and forms the basis of the operation of the instrument known as the GDx (the GDx Access is the model used in modern practices).

The retinal nerve fiber layer shows birefringence of an incident laser and the influence that it has upon the incident confocal laser beam from the instrument is interpreted to infer the thickness of the layer. This results in the nerve fiber layer thickness profiles shown in the Figure 10.3.

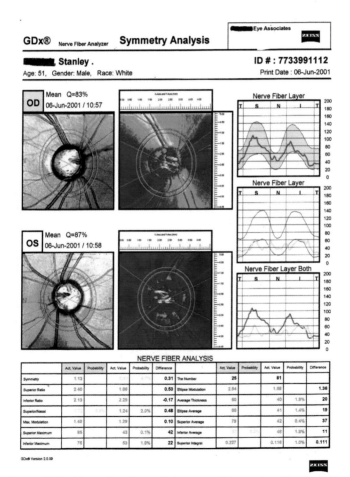

Figure 10.3 Nerve fiber layer thickness profiles produced by the GDx (reproduced with permission from Zeiss)

Because the assessment is made with measurement compared to a reference plane, the technique is not affected by refractive error.

As might be expected, one problem in the development of such a technique has been that birefringence occurs as light passes through the cornea and this must be compensated for if an accurate assessment of the nerve fiber layer is to be achieved. The GDx and GDx Access include such a compensator and this is usually set at a default appropriate for a standard cornea (an 80% setting is typical). If the compensation is not accurate, this may be predicted by unusual data that are not borne out by other assessment.

Much has been published in recent years concerning the accuracy of the GDx unit and nerve fiber analysis. The fact that changes to the NFL may be a useful early indicator of glaucomatous change is well-established and many ophthalmologists have for years used bright or red-free light assessment of the peripapillary area to look for deviations in the way the nerve fibers reflect light. A wedge-shaped area of less reflection would, for example, be treated as suspicious.

The use of NFL analysis as a tool in the effective screening of glaucoma has been found to have a high sensitivity and specificity. More recently, the use of data about the superior to nasal and the inferior to nasal NFL data ratios has been confirmed as effective and sensitive in differentiating between glaucomatous and nonglaucomatous eyes.

There is also evidence to confirm NFL differences may be demonstrated in the eyes of ocular hypertensives. When the technique was assessed to determine its diagnostic accuracy, one study has found that it was effective at differentiating between normal patients and those with glaucomatous damage. However, even the best algorithm tested failed to detect a substantial number of subjects with severe damage.

Bearing this in mind, it seems as if the GDx provides a useful screening assessment of the NFL which makes it potentially valuable to an optometrist wanting a sensitive indicator of potential for glaucoma. It is also useful for monitoring glaucomatous NFL changes over a period of time. It does not, however, replace accurate disk analysis nor does it remove the need for pressures and fields to be monitored.

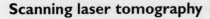

Scanning laser tomography

The accuracy of observation of an ocular structure, such as the optic disc, will be related to the skill and experience of the observer. Accurate photography of the disc allows a more accurate quantitative measurement of two-dimensional data, but the ability to accurately represent a three-dimensional model of the disk is yet more valuable. An instrument which might somehow store an accurate three-dimensional representation of the disk architecture could usefully detect any parameters which are outside an expected norm and would also be able to detect accurately any changes to the disk over a period of time.

When the Heidelberg Retinal Tomograph (HRT) was introduced in 1991, it was described as 'the first scanning laser system for routine glaucoma exam'. Its cost and bulky size proved prohibitive to eye care professionals in general practice, but as a hospital-based research tool able to analyze and store accurate topographic information, it formed the basis of multiple research papers. Topographical analysis using a confocal technique, of course, meant the HRT was useful not only in glaucoma research but also in the investigation of other structural change diseases such as macular holes, macular edema, retinal detachments and neoplasms. There was also some application in the investigation of the atrophic changes in non-exudative macular degeneration.

In effect, the laser is focused and scanned rapidly across a common plane running through the optic nerve head. Elevation or depression of the optic disc relative to this flat plane is measured so allowing an accurate topographic representation of the head to be stored. The software may then predict whether the topography is normal or suspicious of glaucoma, and sequential assessment of a disk over a time period may very sensitively detect changes in disk topography as would occur with a chronic optic neuropathy.

In 1998 a team at Moorfields Eye Hospital completed a study which aimed to define the HRT parameters that best allow it to separate patients with early glaucoma from normal subjects. A total of 131 patients were examined, 51 of whom had glaucoma leading to field loss (averaging a mean deviation of −3.6 dB). Data were taken from the normals regarding the relationship between the neuroretinal rim area and the optic disc area, and the cup/disc ratio and the optic disc area. The normal ranges for these two parameters were defined mathematically (in terms of the 99% prediction intervals of the linear regression between the parameter and the optic disc area) for the whole disc and for each of six predefined segments of disc. It was found that a high sensitivity (96.3%) and specificity (84.3%) in separating the normals from the glaucoma patients was achieved, and that the technique of linear regression provided a good separation method, the best figures being found when the log of the area of the neuroretinal rim was compared to the optic disc area.

A year later the same team published a study with the aim of trying to determine if an analysis of sequential optic disc images using the HRT would be able to demonstrate disk changes in ocular hypertensives before the development of reproducible field defects. They found that there was evidence of disc data recorded by the HRT showing changes over a 1 year period before any field loss was established. This suggested the machine might usefully play a role in glaucoma detection in an at-risk group prior to any field loss.

The HRT II was introduced in 1999 with the aim of providing the benefits of accurate laser scanning techniques in a more clinically friendly form and the instrument itself is similar to a small table-mounted slit-lamp unit with a separate computer and monitor (Figure 10.4). The basic unit itself can he dismantled easily and hence is readily portable.

It is marketed as an instrument for aiding the early detection and the monitoring of glaucoma. However, adapted software is available for analysis of macular edema, retinal analysis and corneal analysis (see below). The instrument contains a diode laser emitting at a wavelength of 670 nm (class 1 laser). The spread allows a field of view of 15° to be analyzed.

Figure 10.5 shows a reading taken from a diagnosed glaucoma patient. The six red crosses clearly demonstrate that the disk profile falls outside the expected norm in all six sectors.

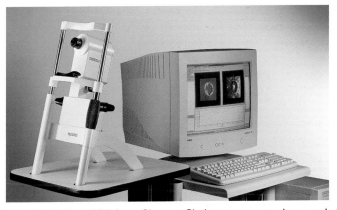

Figure 10.4 The HRTII from Clement Clarke may come to be regarded as an essential instrument for screening for glaucoma, particularly in shared or managed care schemes (reproduced with permission from Doshi & Harvey *Investigative Techniques and Ocular Examination*, Butterworth-Heinemann 2003)

Optical coherence topography

As far back as 1878, Albert Michelson hypothesized that, if it were possible to split a beam of light into two parts and then transmit them along perpendicular paths, it might be possible upon receiving the returning beams to detect any differences in phase between them. This difference or interference would give valuable data about the surfaces from which the light has been reflected. This was the basis of the Michelson Interferometer, and is now the basis of the Zeiss Stratus OCT (Figure 10.6).

In this instrument, a light beam is sent simultaneously to the eye and a reference mirror. The light penetrates through retinal tissues ad is reflected back. The returning light is compared to the reference and this allows software to reconstruct a representation of the underlying tissues. This ability to, in effect, show a cross-section through retina makes the machine invaluable in monitoring lesions such as the macular hole shown in Figure 10.7.

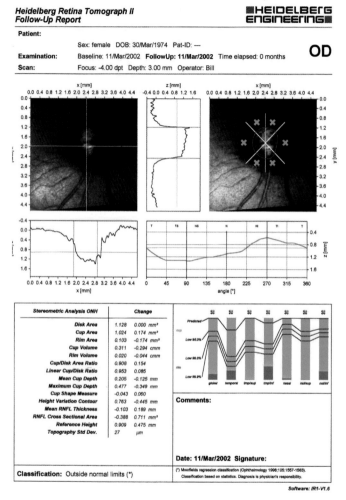

Figure 10.5 Reading taken from a diagnosed glaucoma patient. HRT II data

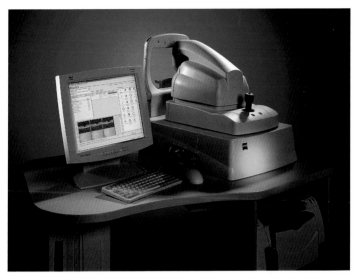

Figure 10.6 Zeiss Stratus OCT

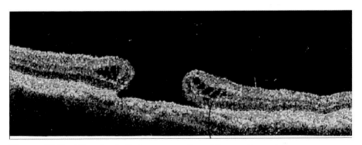

Figure 10.7 Macular hole image produced by ocular coherence
tomography

Anterior confocal microscopy

Confocal microscopy has been a familiar technique in university
and hospital research departments, allowing a practitioner to
carry out cell counts, and monitor minor structural changes.
Such work on the endothelium is the basis of much of our
knowledge about how this structure changes with age or with

external insult (such as hypoxic stress) and much significant knowledge has been gained. Other research, such as looking at the effects of topical therapeutic agents, contact lenses and developmental variations may all be assessed in vivo with a significant advantage over in vitro techniques.

Like many other areas of optometric technology, the advances in refractive surgery have led to an increased demand for good resolution yet easy to achieve confocal corneal images. One of the best indications of postoperative corneal recovery (either for a photorefractive treatment such as Lasik or phototherapeutic intervention such as graft surgery) is to look for changes to cellular structure within the cornea, or to visualize debris build-up. For example, a high-resolution confocal view of the stroma post-Lasik may allow changes to the keratocytes to be detected, as well as increases in cell debris or corneal nerve changes. Doing this at intervals after surgery gives an excellent indication of corneal recovery and is an integral part of most refractive surgeons' follow-up routine.

The technique also has a more noniatrogenic use, however, in the detection and monitoring of corneal disease. For example, the Langerhans cell population in the plane of the basal cell layer near the limbus is useful in assessing the keratoconic, particularly after a full-thickness graft. Cellular changes and guttata may be detected at an early stage in Fuch's dystrophy. Microcystic response, either related to hypoxic insult or keratitis, may be monitored with much greater accuracy than a slit-lamp would afford. It is even possible to analyze erythrocyte flow in a neovascular response. Furthermore, the increasing use of mitomycin drugs in corneal recovery may be monitored. In summary, the confocal microscope adds an extra dimension to corneal assessment over and beyond the slit-lamp and, as such, is an increasingly important tool in the armory of any corneal or contact lens specialist, either optometric or ophthalmologic. An extra benefit to being able to focus on any plane in the cornea is the ability to accurately assess corneal thickness. The distance between the confocal planes imaged at the front and back surfaces of the cornea provides this information.

Recently, an adapter to the HRT II (see earlier) allows the confocal laser previously focused in the plane of the optic disc to instead be focused at the cornea so providing a useful image of any plane throughout the cornea.

Topographers

In 1847 the English physician Henry Goode used the reflection of a square target from the cornea to decide upon corneal shape in what is claimed to be the first keratoscope. Independently, in 1880 the Portuguese oculist Antonio Placido introduced the now famous black and white concentric ring target with a viewing hole to analyze the distortion of the reflected rings from the cornea; the first photokeratoscope. It is a variation of the Placido's disk which is the basis of most modern computerized topographers. At this stage, assessment of corneal contour was primarily qualitative, with subjective assessment being made of distortion of the reflected image. The introduction of computer analysis of the reflected targets, which began in earnest in the late 1980s, allowed the development of the quantification of reflected image changes. By sampling changes to the image at many points, a very accurate profile of the corneal contour may be constructed, and then represented in a variety of representations or 'maps'.

The various maps are usually color coded; red areas show where the cornea is steepest and blue areas where it is flatter (Figure 10.8). Difference maps may allow a change in profile, for example after contact lens wear, to be shown.

More recent topographers, such as the Orbscan, use a slit-beam scanning device which allows not only the anterior corneal surface profile to be measured, but also the posterior surface. Furthermore, topographers may also represent the tear profile underneath a contact lens, so providing a useful alternative to the far more subjective fluorescein assessment.

The increasing use of topographers in contact lens practice has led to some software to generate the ideal contact lens parameter for corneal fitting. It is also the basis of the resurgence in popularity of orthokeratology, where the deliberate remolding of the cornea

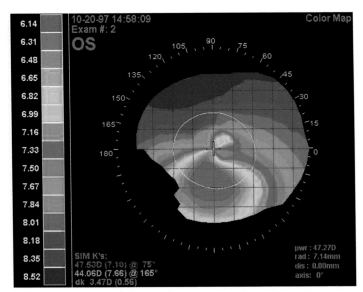

Figure 10.8 Topography – color-coded map. Note cooler colors indicate flatter areas, warmer colors are steeper

by selective lens fitting to overcome refractive error, where vastly improved accuracy and predictability has been made possible.

The increased use of topographers as part of the preoperative assessment before refractive surgery has also resulted in increasing numbers of early corneal dystrophies, such as keratoconus, to be detected. This shows that the machines have a diagnostic as well as a biometric role.

Aberrometry

When describing the very great amount of aberration that affects light passing through the human eye, Helmholtz once remarked 'If an optician wanted to sell me an instrument which had all these defects . . . I should give him back his instrument'. Refractive correction may compensate for the so-called lower-order aberrations, but the final image is reduced by an array of higher-order aberrations. The impact of these may be measured using an aberrometer. This relies upon an analysis of how a wavefront passing through the eye is altered. If the eye is aberration free, then an incident plane wave will be refracted to form a regular wave. The eye, however, is not aberration free and hence the resultant wave is distorted (Figure 10.9a,b). It is

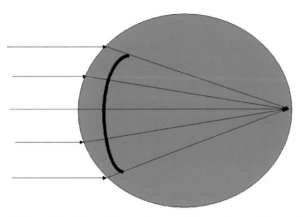

Figure 10.9a Parallel rays from a distant object are focused at a point in an eye without aberrations

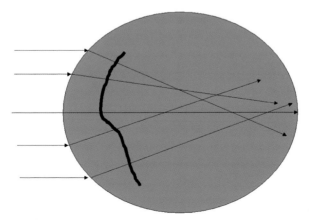

Figure 10.9b Parallel rays from a distant object are focussed at various retinal positions in an eye with aberrations

possible to measure the change from the regular wave at many points so recording the wavefront aberration. Most aberrometers use a system called the Hartmann–Shack. This employs an array of tiny lenses (lenslets) through which the aberrant wavefront passes. Each lenslet forms a point image which would be a perfect point for each were the wavefront to be aberration free. However, the point spread at each point focus reveals the overall aberration. The accurate analysis of this gives useful information which may be used, for example, in programing the laser used in refractive surgery such that the postoperative corneal profile has less aberrations, or in specifying contact lens design with minimal aberration for the cornea to which it is to be fitted.

Further reading

American Academy of Ophthalmology (1996) *Preferred Practice Pattern: Primary Open Angle Glaucoma* American Academy of Ophthalmology: San Francisco.

Index